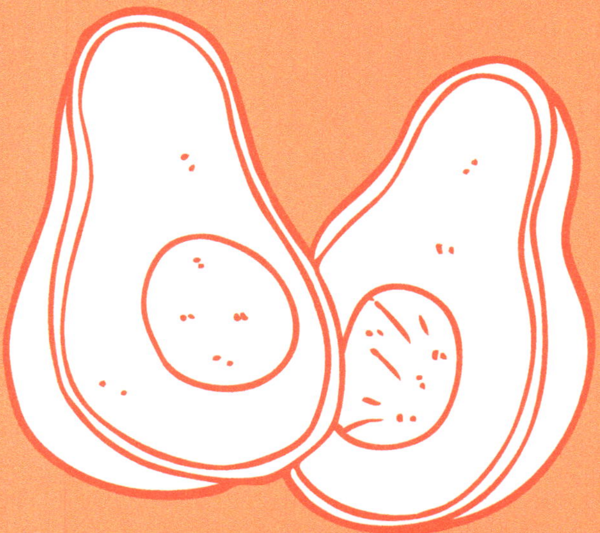

This workbook belongs to:

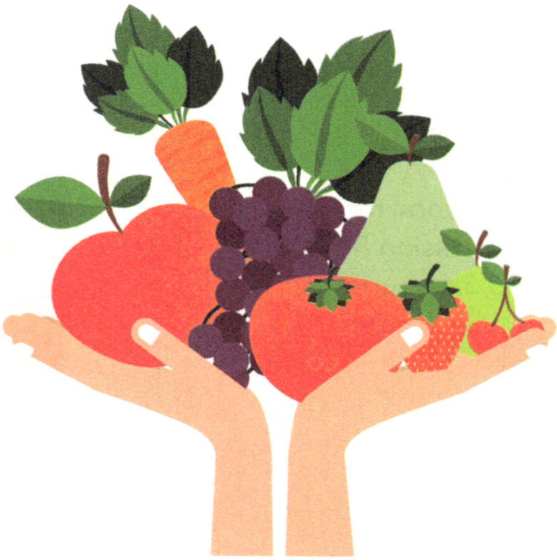

FRUITS & VEGETABLES

Learn the Alphabet and COLORS Nutrition Workbook

Ages 3-4

Lexi Striler, RD and Tammy Striler, M.S. Ed.

For permissions contact: hello@healthnhoney.co

Striler Publishing
healthnhoney.co

Title: Learn the Alphabet and Colors Nutrition Workbook: Fruits & Vegetables
Authors: Lexi Striler & Tammy Striler
Interior and Cover Designer: Lexi Striler
Author photographic design: Kyra Badiner

Graphics and illustrations used under One Design Use License and Free Media License from Canva.com.

ISBN: [978-0-9828796-8-9] (print)
Printed in the USA
First printing, July 2021

Created in San Diego, California, USA

PARENT GUIDE

The educational benefits behind this workbook!

ABOUT THIS WORKBOOK

Background:

We are a mother-daughter duo who couldn't be more proud of combining our expertise to create this one-of-a-kind learning workbook for children. Lexi, a Registered Dietitian, and Tammy, an elementary school teacher of 30+ years, know that teaching kids about nutrition early on is very beneficial. We developed this educational learn-to-write workbook for kids that emphasizes the healthiest foods you can eat— fruits and vegetables!

Health Benefits:

The foods children are exposed to in their early years play a big role in their lives. This is why we prioritized healthy habits at an early age. The more familiar these foods are to children at a young age, the more willing they are to try new and healthy foods.

From asparagus to zucchini, we highlight produce that is less conventional so your child can see, and ultimately try, more of a variety. It's important to steer away from "ew, broccoli!" to a more neutral and open mind when it comes to the greens (and reds, oranges, purples, etc.) that are on their plate. Have them try some of the tasty recipes that go along with the letters so they can make their own opinions about these fruits and vegetables!

Educational Benefits:

It's important for children to engage in vocabulary with unfamiliar words. You'll notice that we don't always use the most common fruits and vegetables— and that is by design. We want children to see and hear words that they are unfamiliar with so they can build up their own vocabulary and who knows, maybe even try something new!

We made two versions of this workbook: Preschool Edition (ages 3-4) and Early Elementary Edition (ages 5-7). These workbooks are designed to be an interactive learning experience for you and your child— so have fun!

Preschool:

The preschool book emphasizes vocabulary, letter recognition, letter tracing, and colors. Preschoolers need to engage in oral conversations and explore fruits & vegetables through the hands-on learning activities and recipes included in the workbook.

Early Elementary:

The early elementary book emphasizes writing, vocabulary, handwriting, and drawing. The writing section in this book is an important part of learning to write. Whether the child is writing the sentence on their own, or an adult writes it for them, the child is coming up with the content. This is more meaningful because it is their thoughts and ideas— and because they came up with the sentence, they will be excited to “read” it back to you. Their drawing that goes with the sentence is their way of showing the meaning behind it, which is more impactful than just copying a prewritten sentence.

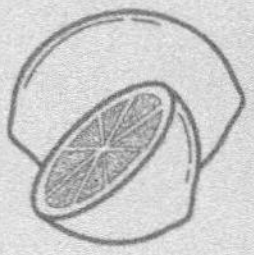

We hope you and your child enjoy this workbook as much as we enjoyed making it!

- Lexi and Tammy

WHAT ARE FRUITS AND VEGETABLES?

Before we learn about all different kinds of fruits and vegetables, let's first define what they are!

To put it simply, fruits and vegetables are classified based on the part of the plant they come from.

FRUITS

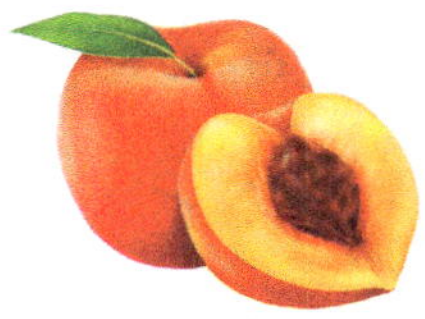

- come from the flower of a plant
- contain seeds

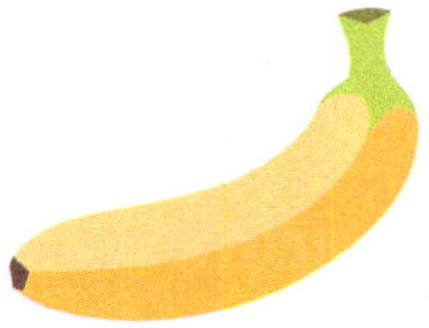

VEGETABLES

- come from any other edible part of a plant

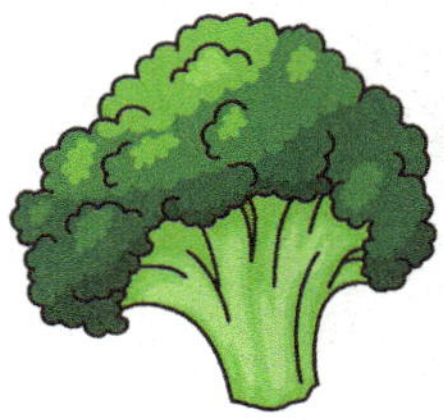

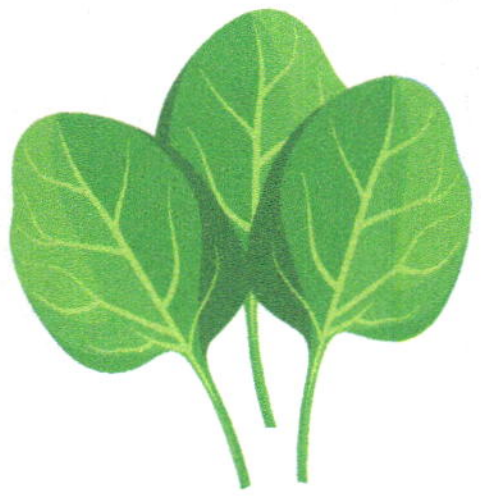

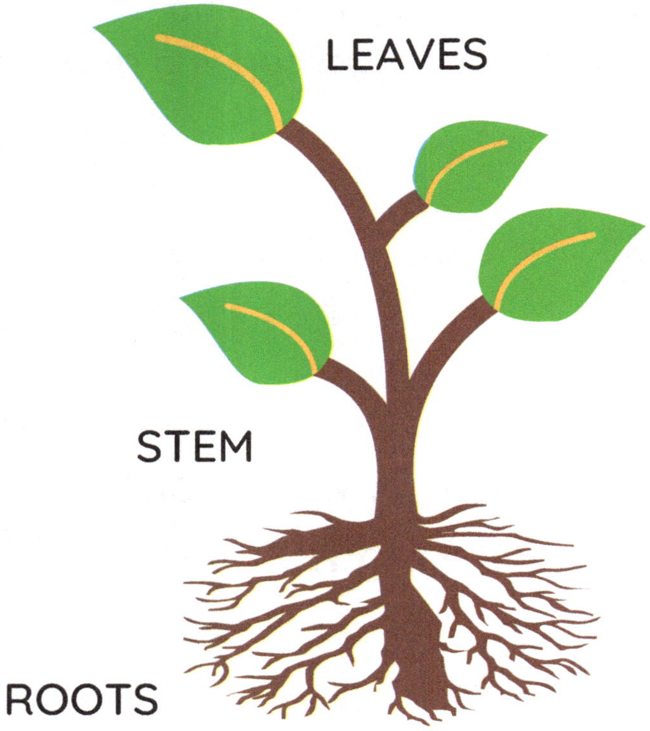

To the left is an example of an edible plant. Vegetables make up different parts of this plant such as the roots (example: carrots), stems (example: celery), or the leaves (example: lettuce).

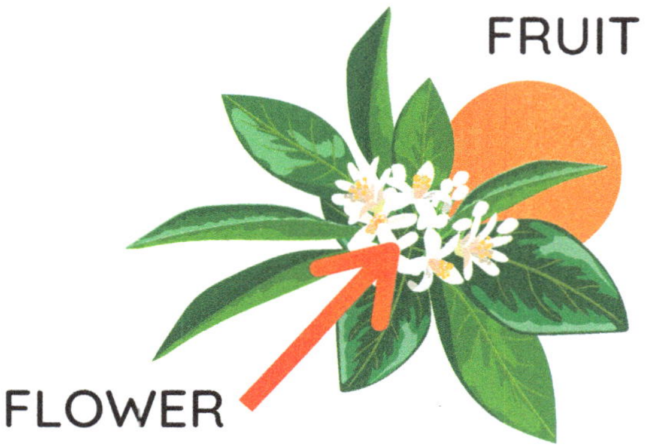

While fruits still grow from a plant, they can only grow from ones that have a flower. This example shows an orange fruit growing out of a flower blossom.

Fruits & Vegetables: Botanically Defined vs. How We Eat Them

The topic of fruits and vegetables can be a little confusing because the botanical definition of fruits and vegetables may be different than how we eat them.

For example, avocados, tomatoes, and zucchini are all botanically fruits because they grow out of flowers and contain seeds. However, we do not eat these as fruits because, in terms of eating, fruits are considered to taste sweet. These examples above are typically eaten as vegetables because they are more savory. For the sake of this book, we will be differentiating fruits and vegetables based on how we eat them rather than how they are botanically defined.

Five Senses

As we learn about various fruits and vegetables, encourage your child to use their senses when discovering new ones. Explore these senses on both raw and cooked fruits and vegetables.

- Sight: Color, size, shape, characteristics (ex: contains peel)
- Touch: Bumpy, smooth, hard, soft, sticky, heavy, gooey, fuzzy
- Smell: Sweet, neutral, citrusy, woody, mild, spicy
- Taste: Sweet, bland, savory, bitter, sour, cool, hot, spicy
- Sound: Crunchy, hollow, rattle (ex: seeds), sizzle (ex: cooking)

INTRODUCING NEW FOODS

Whether your child is more hesitant or enthusiastic to try new foods, these are helpful ways to welcome unfamiliar foods into your child's diet in a neutral and pressure-free way.

Pro Tip: If you think your child is a "picky eater," try not to use this terminology with them as it can impact their perspective on foods. Instead, remember that eating new foods can take time so stay patient with your child during their food journey!

Language Around Foods:

It's important for kids to politely decline foods they don't prefer rather than declare they "hate it." If they constantly tell themselves they dislike a particular food, they are less likely to give it a second chance when they are older. As we know, taste buds can change as we age, so it's important they keep an open mind with foods.

Avoid: "Ew, broccoli" or "I hate broccoli"
Encourage: "I don't like broccoli today", "No thank you", "That's not my taste", or "I don't care for it yet"

Safe Foods

Children are more likely to try a new food if they have a safe (or known) food to eat as well. Whether their safe food is an apple stick or noodles, allow them to first try their safe food before they are encouraged to try a new food. That way if they dislike the new food (which is okay!) they can go back to the food they know they like and are familiar with.

Parent as the Role Model:

When your child is reluctant to try a new food, have them make your plate with that unfamiliar food on it. This allows them to interactively observe you eat new foods while you discuss what you like about it together.

Additional Learning Activities:

The alphabet pages in the workbook can be turned into a hands-on activity so your child can become even more comfortable with new fruits and vegetables, especially if they're not ready to try them yet. In the Learning Activities pages, keep an eye out for the "**bonus activities**" we designed to expose your picky eater to new foods using their senses. After all, exposure is key!

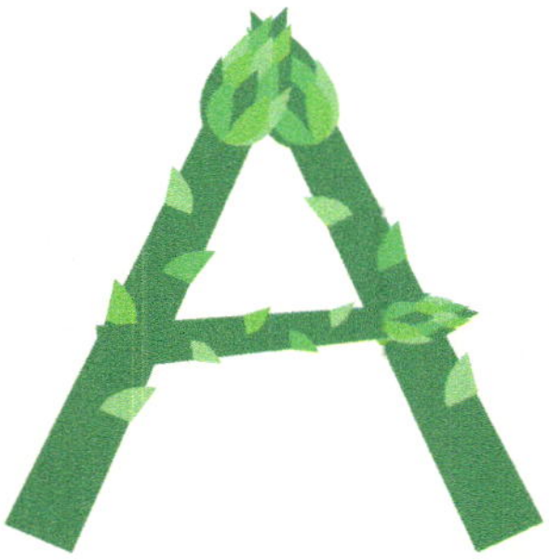

Make the Letter

Make the letter out of the respective fruit or vegetable that starts with that specific letter. For example, if focusing on the letter 'A', have your child make the letter out of asparagus stalks. While doing so, encourage them to explore the five senses. What does this fruit or vegetable look like? Does it have a smell? What texture is it? If they're open to it, have them take a lick or bite. What does it taste like?

"Paint" the Letter

With a fresh painter's palette, fill each cubby with a different dip that your child likes. The dips become the "paints." Pick a letter from the alphabet and have your child "paint" the letter with the fruit or vegetable that begins with that same letter. For example, if the letter is 'B', your child will paint this letter on a clean plate with a piece of broccoli. This helps familiarize them with the food without the pressure of eating it. However, if they do want to munch on it as a snack, that's a bonus!

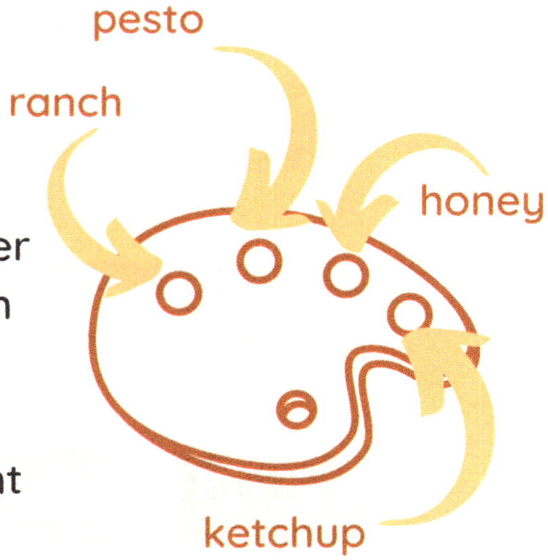

References: Feeding Littles (feedinglittles.com) and "Picky Eater Strategy: Muffin Tin Tapas" by Jenny Rosenstrach (https://cupofjo.com/2019/07/picky-eater-muffin-tin-dinner/). Be sure to check them out for additional resources! Other helpful resources include Solid Starts, Real Mom Nutrition, and Jill Castle, MS, RD.

LEARN THE COLORS

Have these crayons ready for the activities!

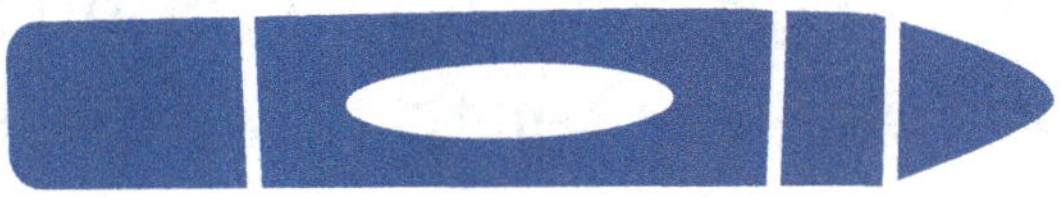

BLUE

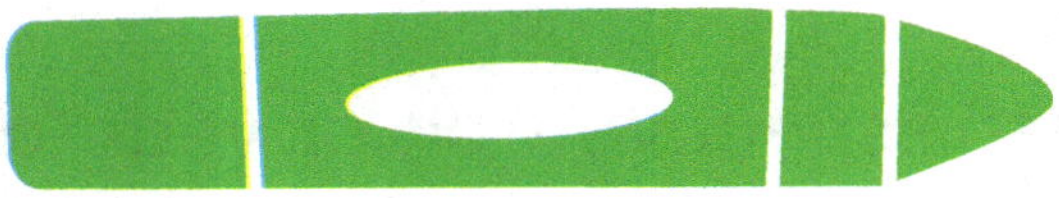

GREEN

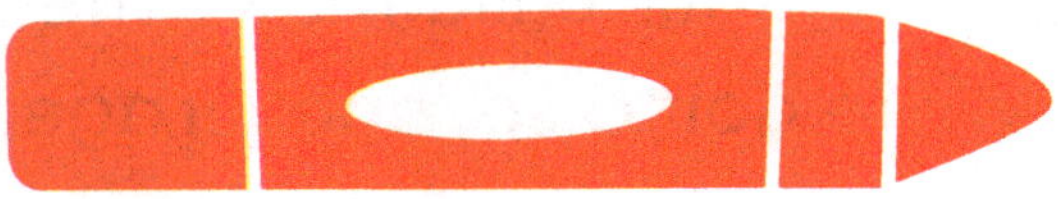

RED

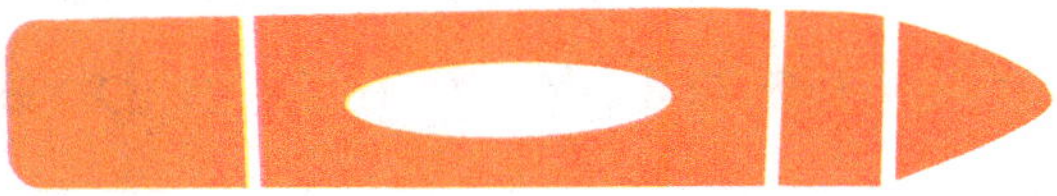

ORANGE

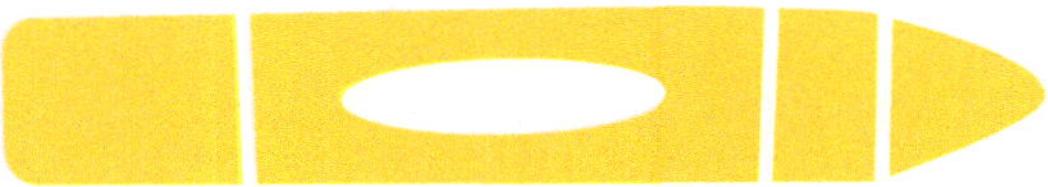

YELLOW

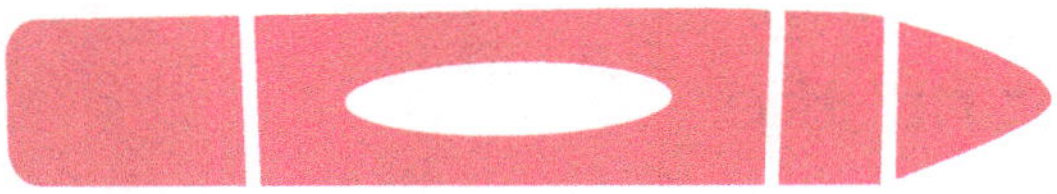

PINK

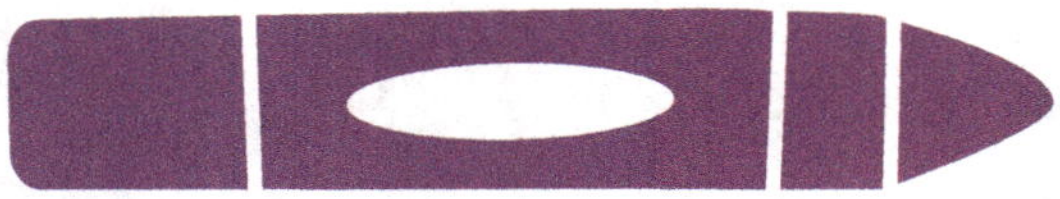

PURPLE

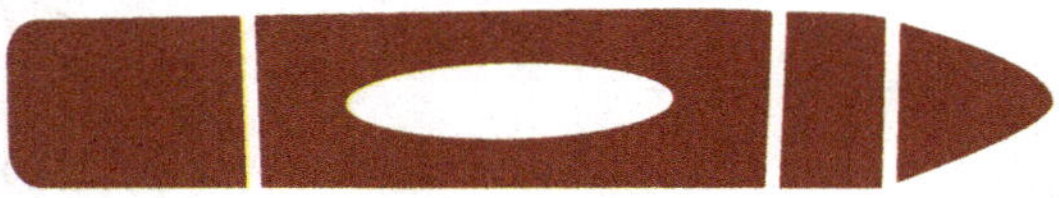

BROWN

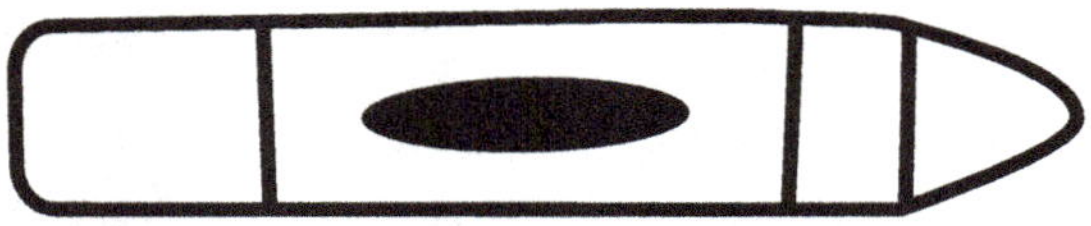

WHITE

Aa

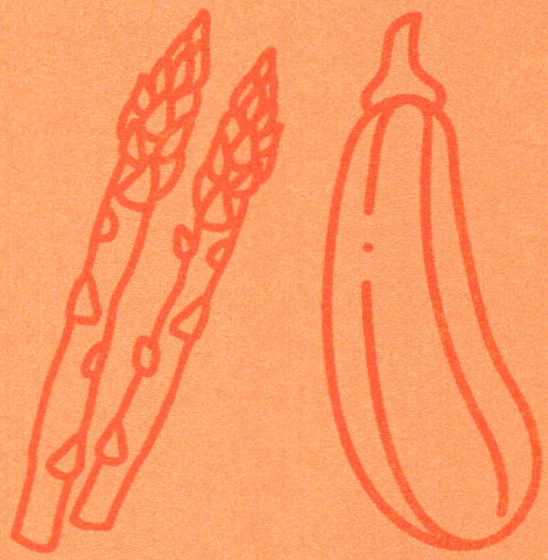

LEARNING THE ALPHABET

Zz

A

ASPARAGUS

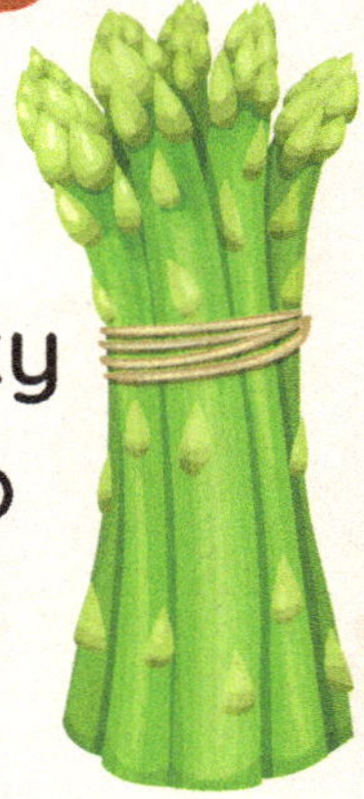

Fun fact: From seed to harvest, it takes this stalky vegetable three years to grow big enough to eat!

Recipe in back of book!

Directions: Color the 'a' fruits and vegetables.

Fruit: apricot	Vegetable: artichoke
Color me ORANGE	Color me GREEN
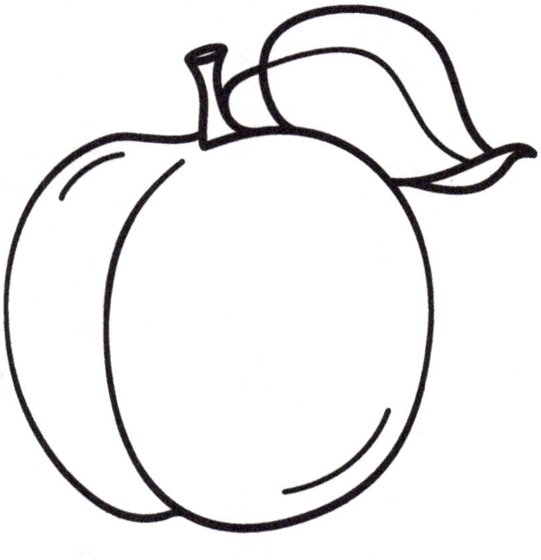	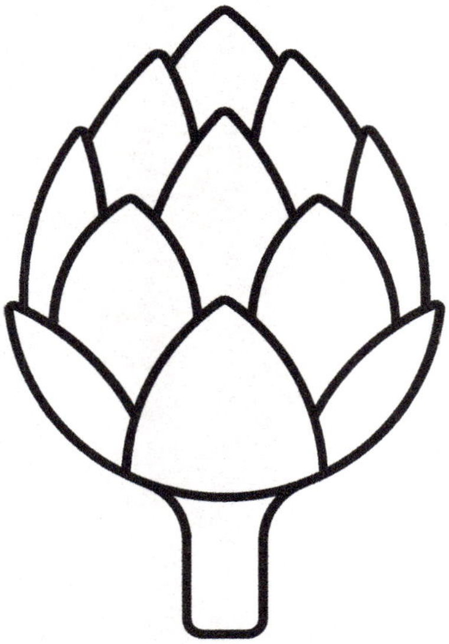

Trace & color me

GREEN

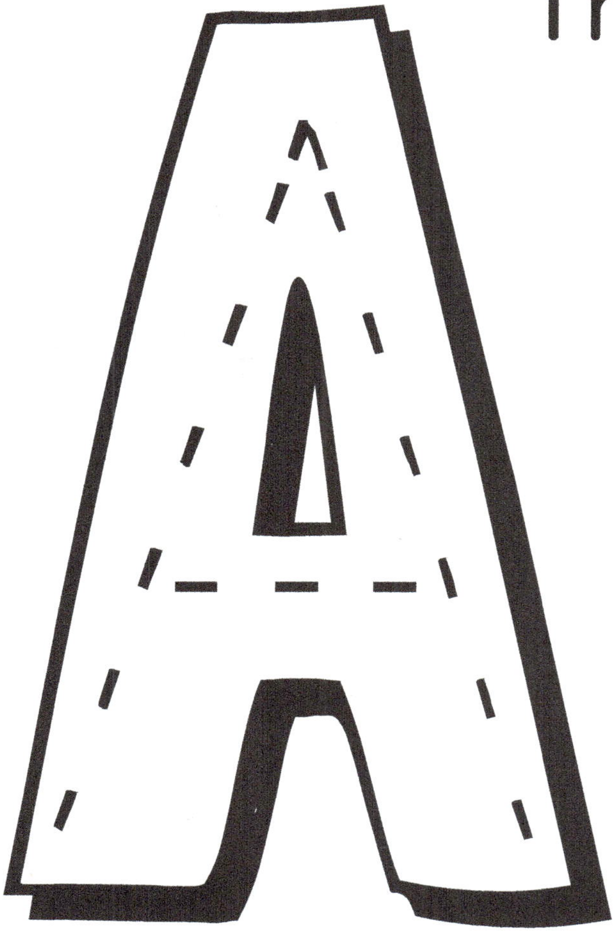

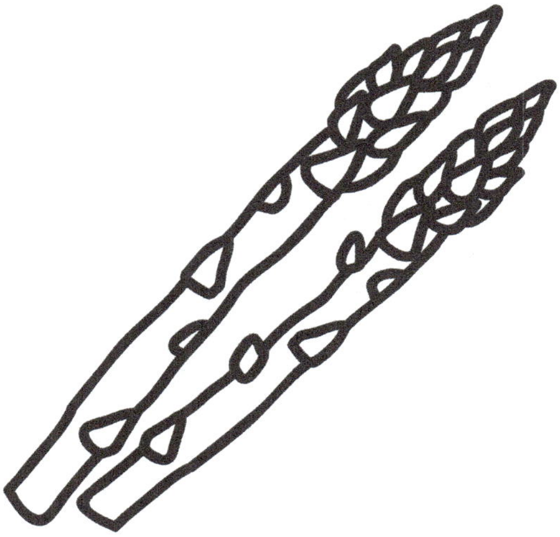

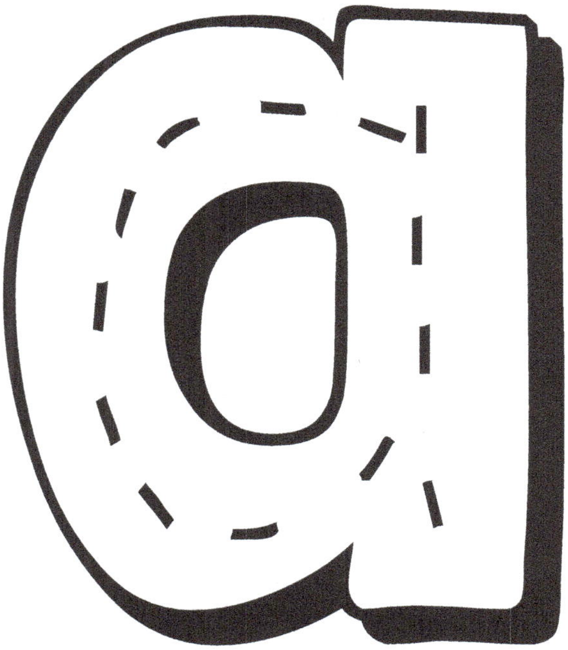

B

BLUEBERRY

A superfruit that helps your body fight off icky sicknesses.

Recipe in back of book!

Directions: Color the 'b' fruits and vegetables.

Fruit:	Vegetable:
banana	broccoli
Color me YELLOW	Color me GREEN
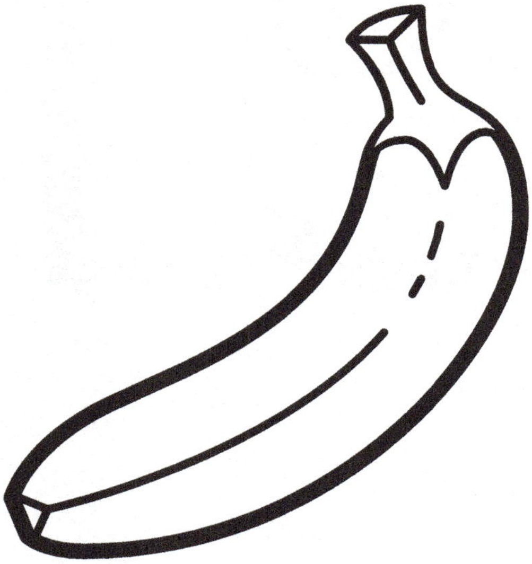	

Trace & color me

BLUE

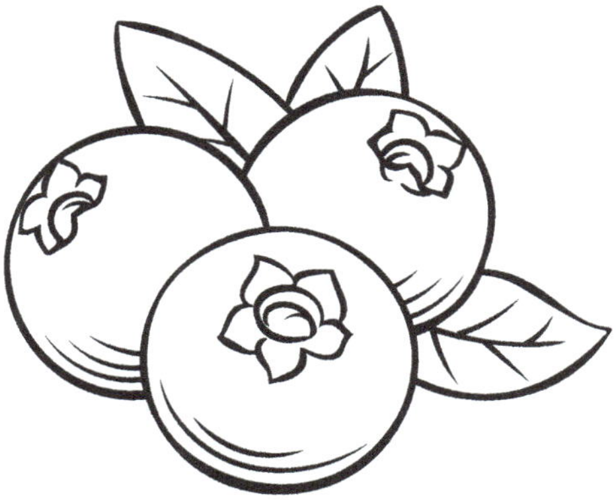

Bb

C

CELERY

This crunchy vegetable is a perfect snack that you can enjoy with savory or sweet dips!

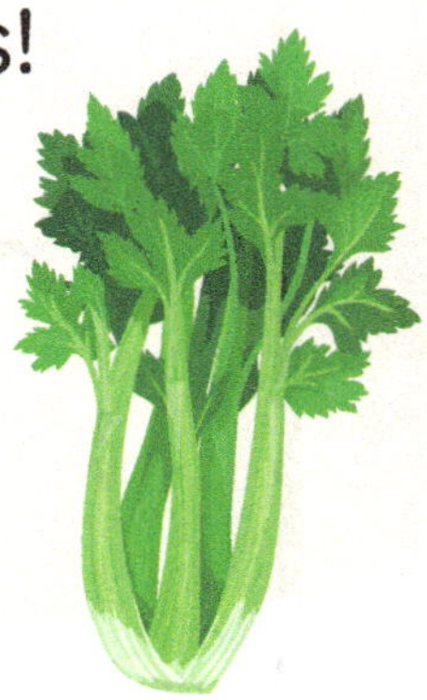

Recipe in back of book!

Directions: Color the 'c' fruits and vegetables.

Fruit: cherry	Vegetable: cauliflower
Color me RED	Color me WHITE
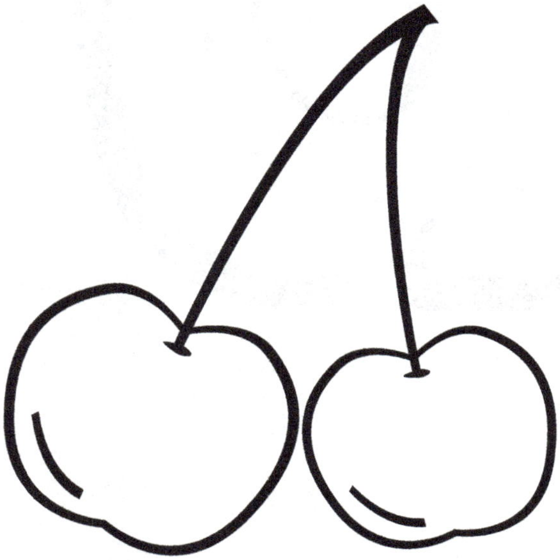	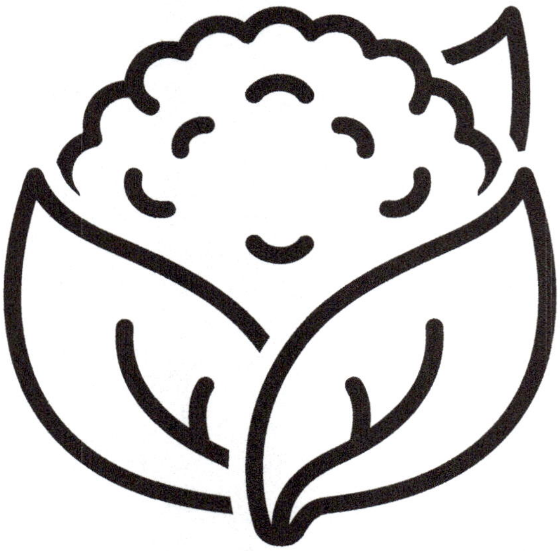

Trace & color me

GREEN

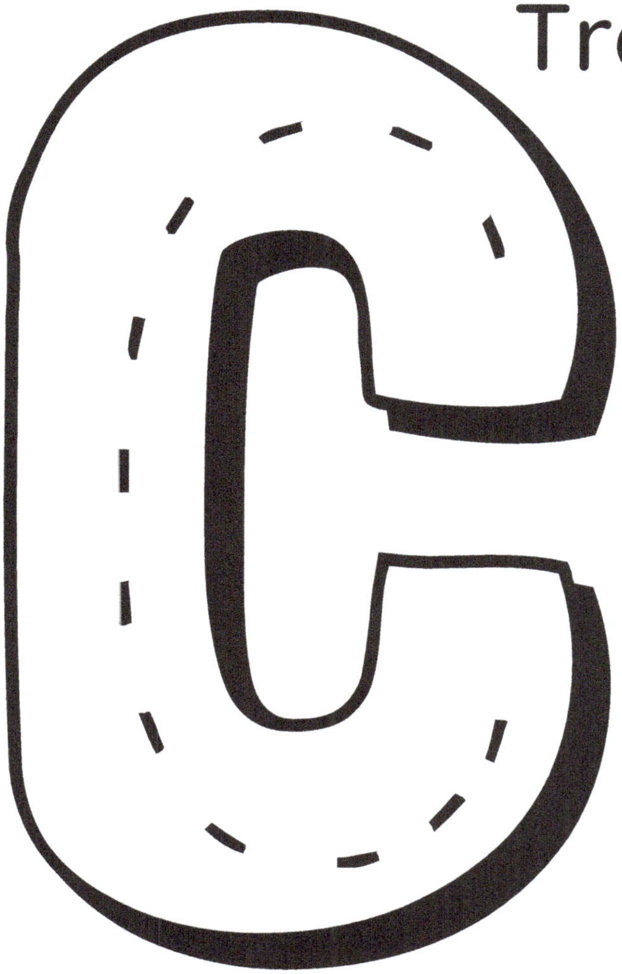

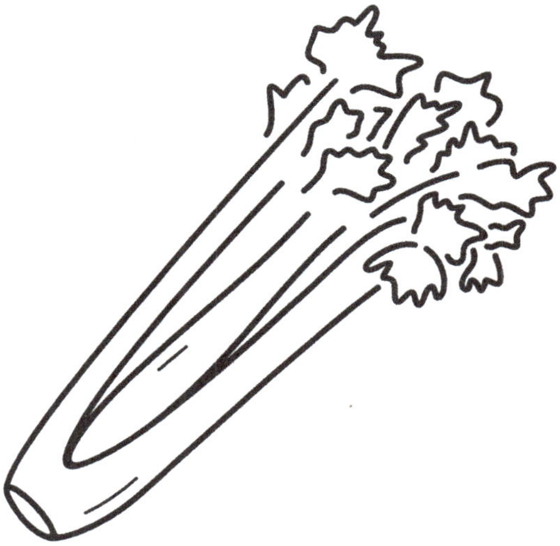

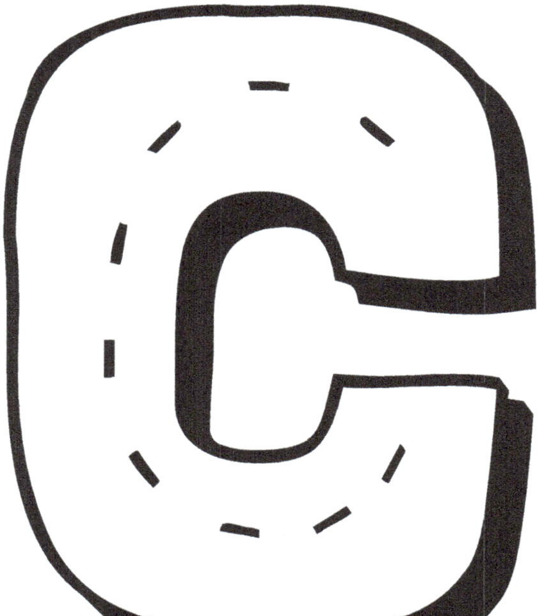

D

DATE

These fruits are healthy and as sweet as candy. You can eat them fresh or even dried!

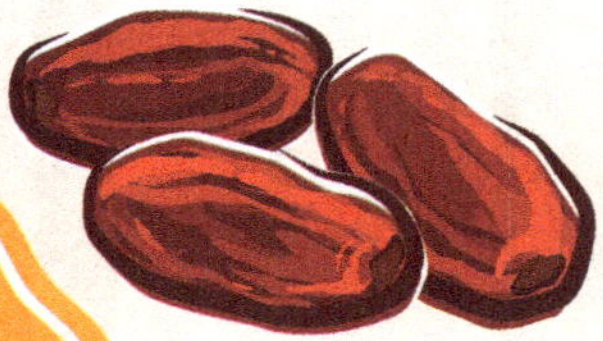

Recipe in back of book!

Directions: Color the 'd' fruits and vegetables.

Fruit:
dragon fruit

Color me PINK

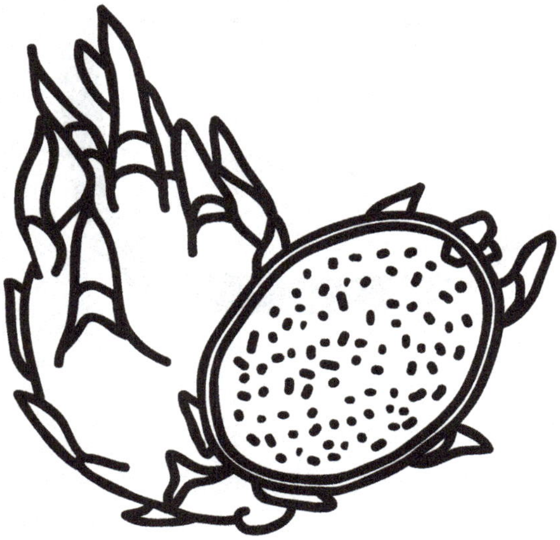

Vegetable:
dried tomato

Color me RED

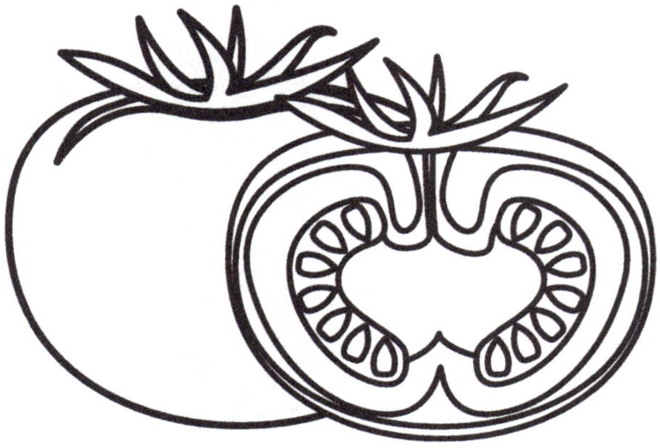

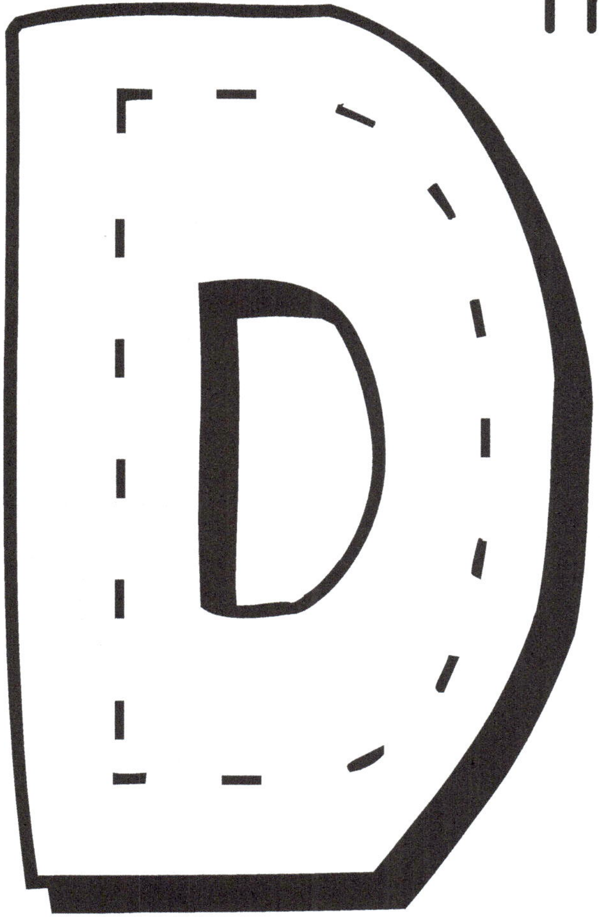

Trace & color me

BROWN

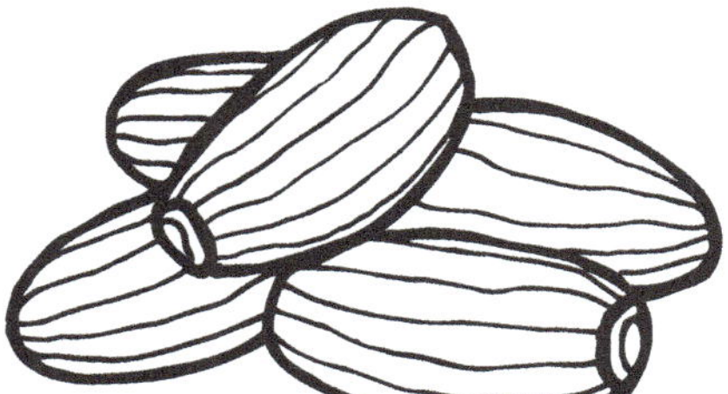

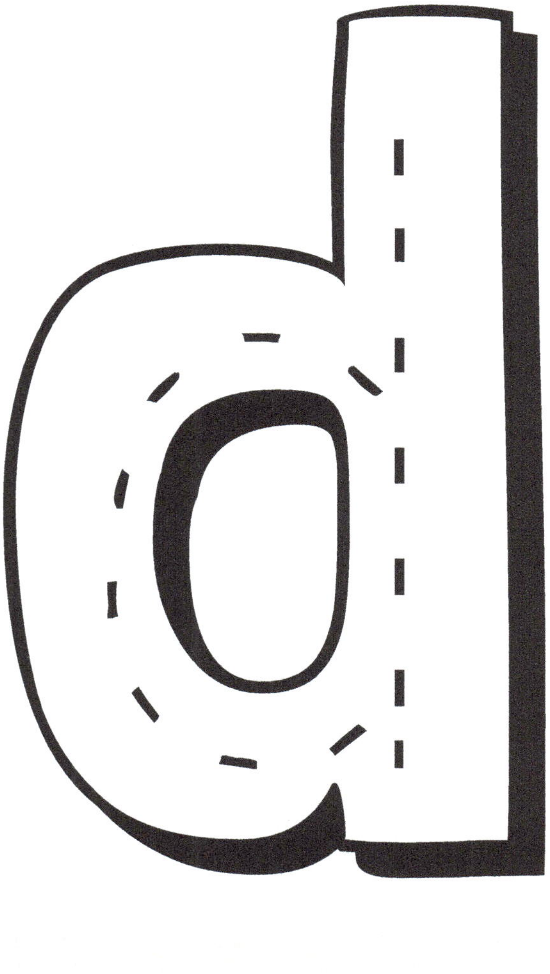

E

EGGPLANT

This purple vegetable is typically cooked into savory dishes. However, did you know that it is technically part of the berry family?

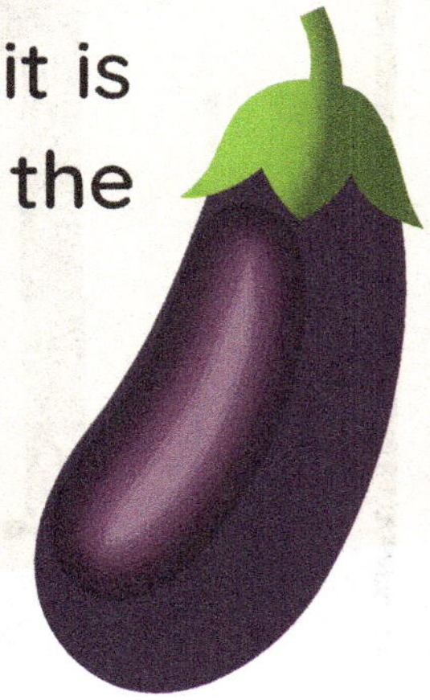

Directions: Color the 'e' fruits and vegetables.

Fruit: elderberry	Vegetable: edamame
Color me BLUE	Color me GREEN
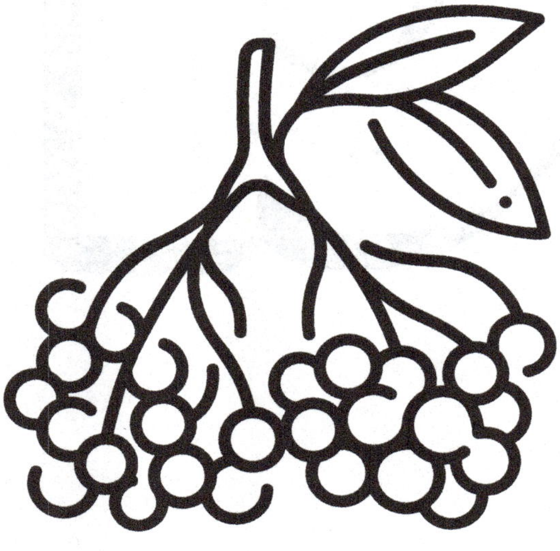	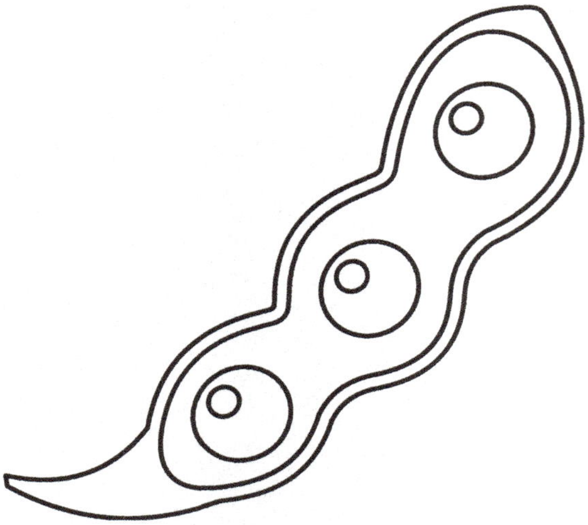

Trace & color me

PURPLE

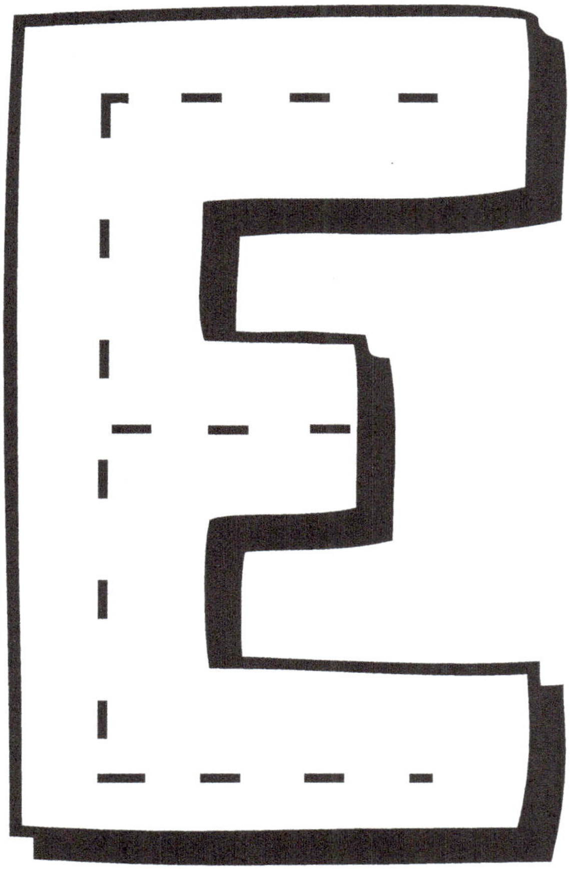

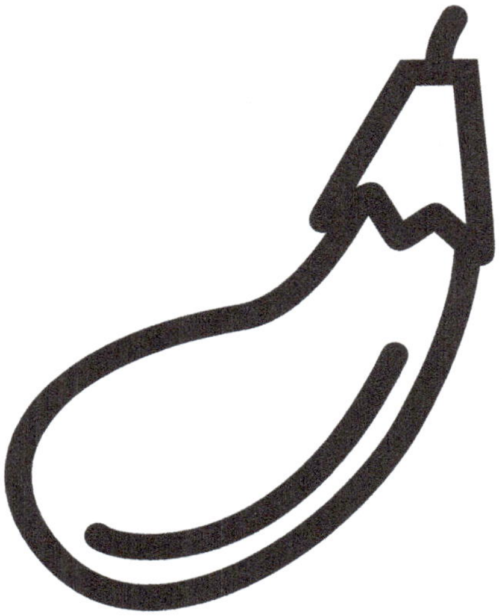

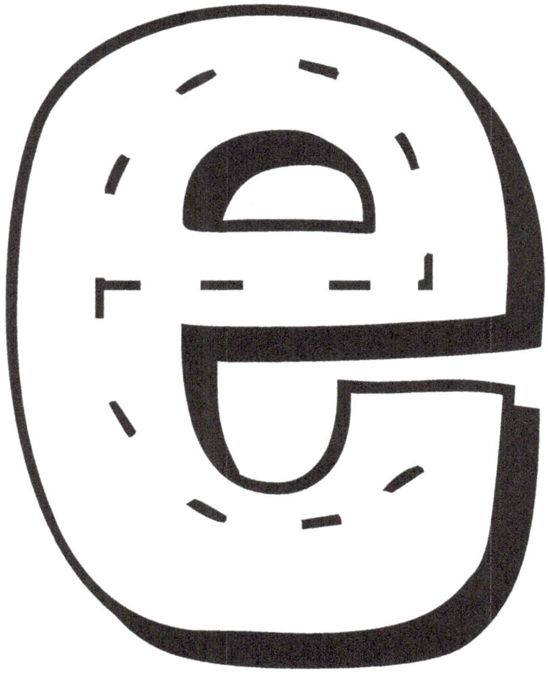

F

FIG

Use figs in your baked goods to sweeten them up in a healthy way!

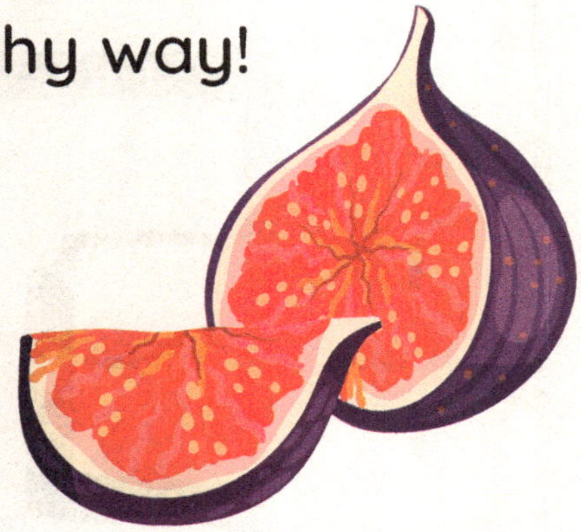

Directions: Color the 'f' fruits and vegetables.

Fruit: Fuji apple **Color me RED**	**Vegetable:** fennel **Color me GREEN**
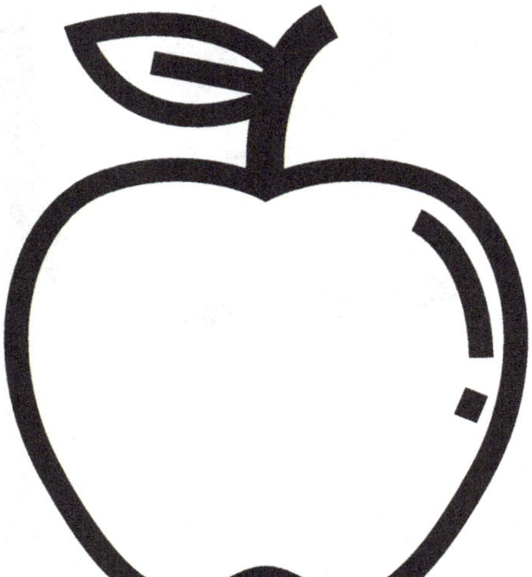	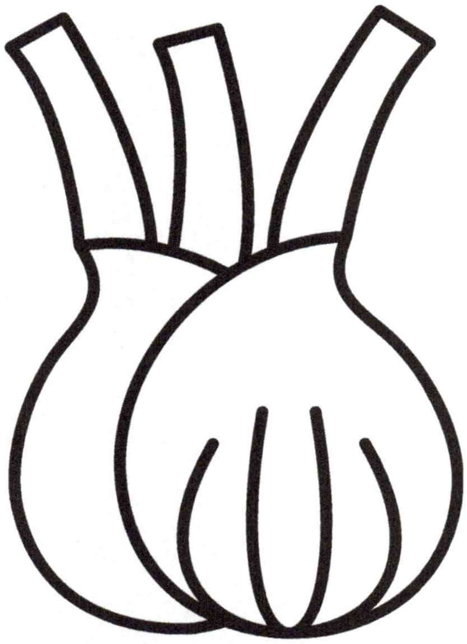

Trace & color me

PINK + PURPLE

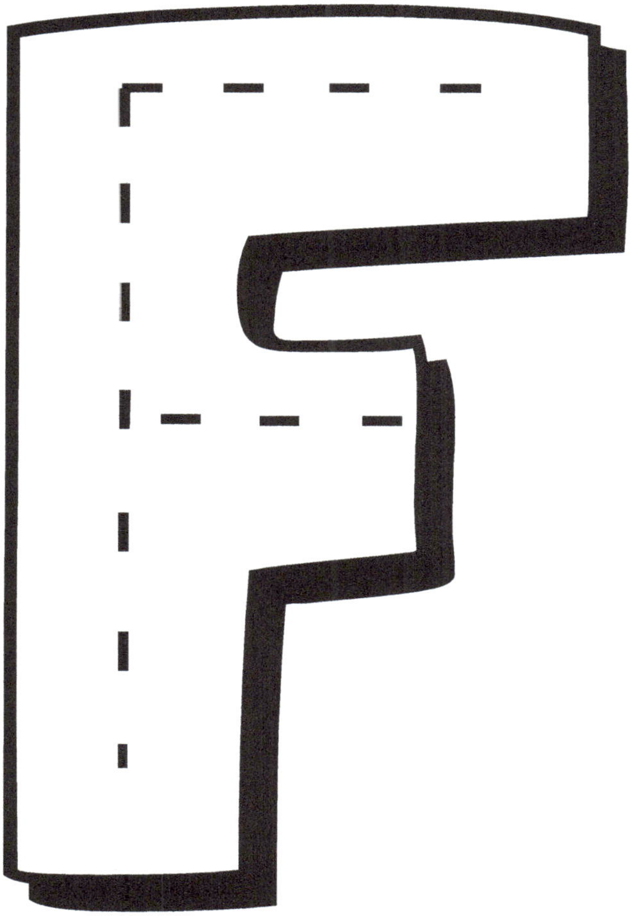

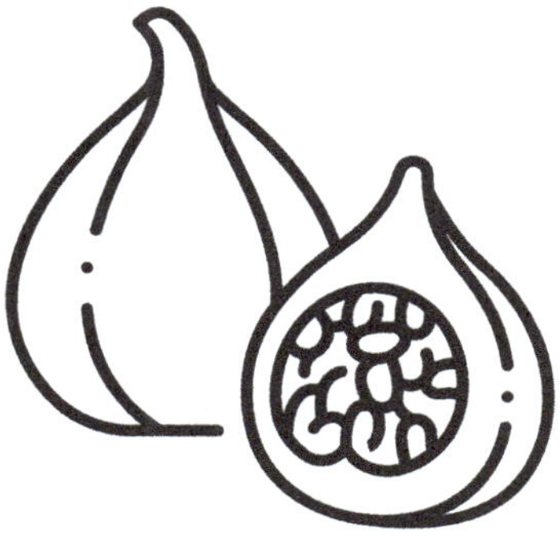

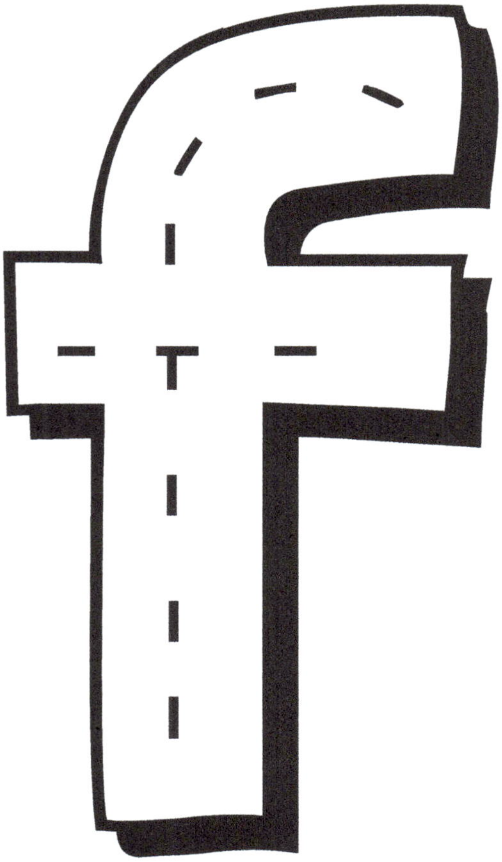

G

GUAVA

Add this tropical fruit to your smoothies by using frozen guava or guava juice!

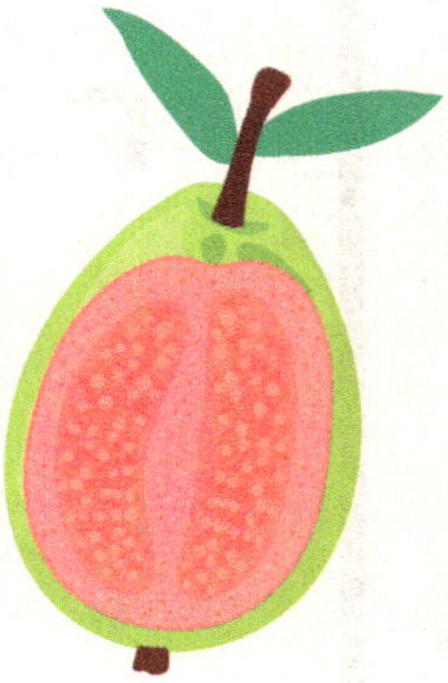

Directions: Color the 'g' fruits and vegetables.

Fruit:
grapefruit

Color me YELLOW

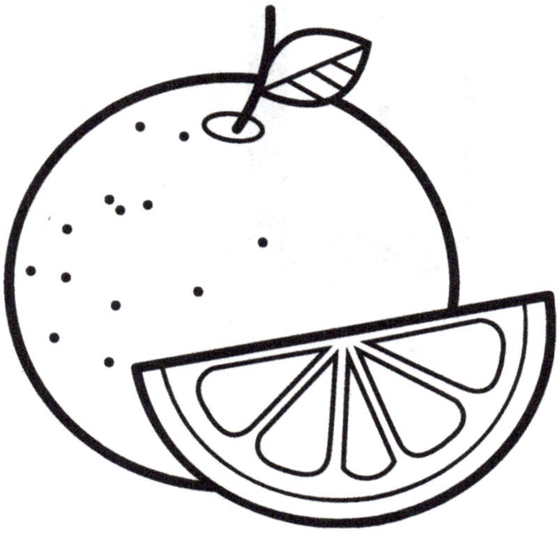

Vegetable:
green bean

Color me GREEN

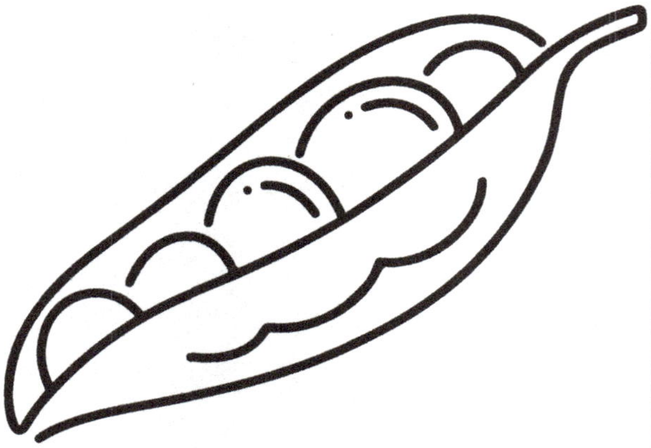

Trace & color me

GREEN + PINK

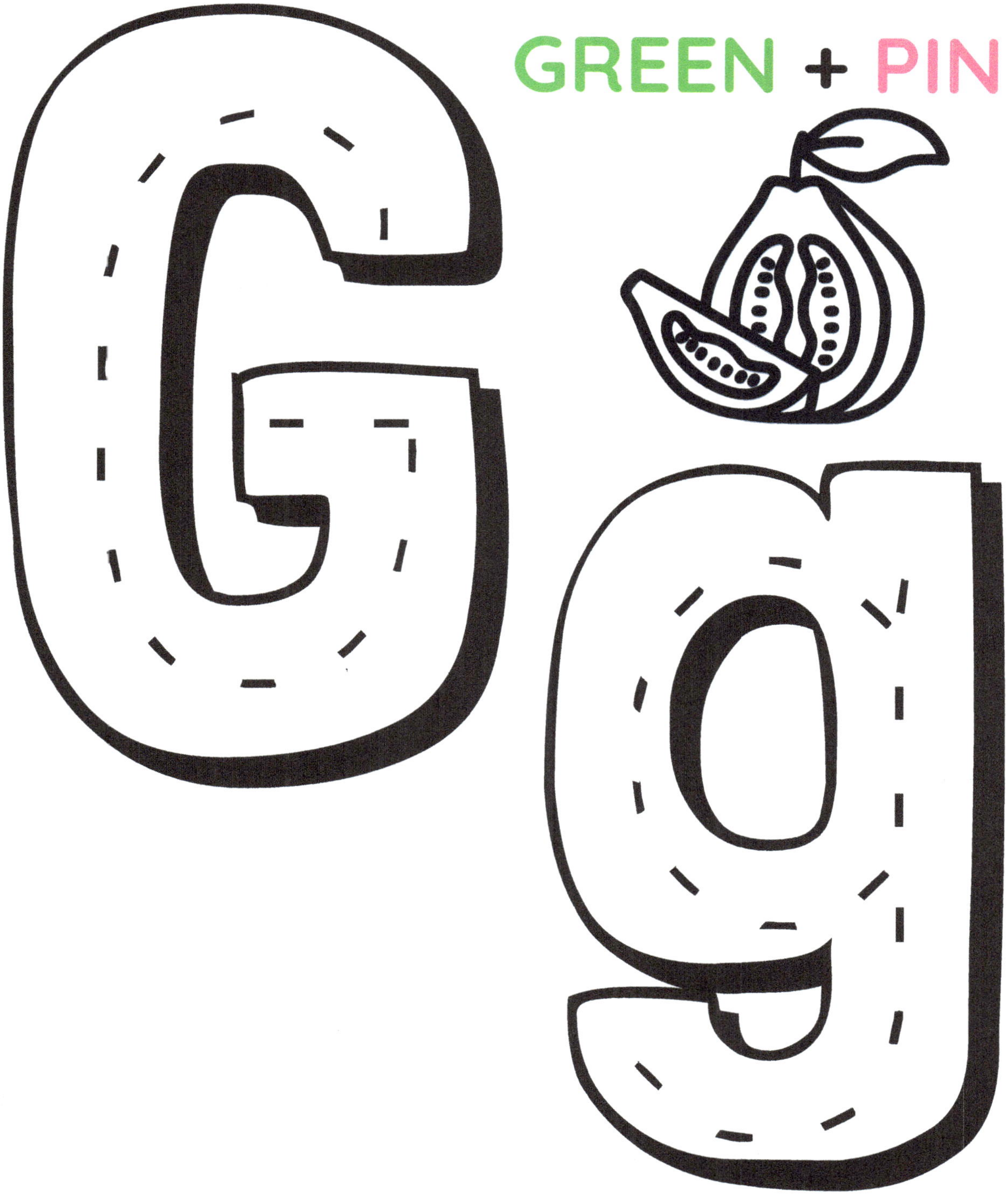

H

HONEYDEW

Fun fact: This fruit is the sweetest of all melons and is related to squash and cucumbers!

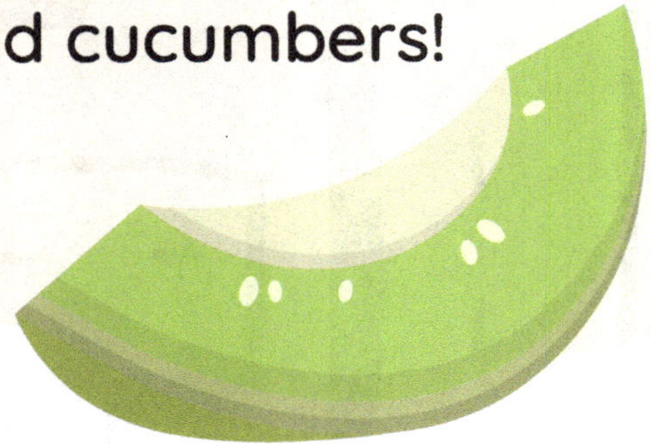

Directions: Color the 'h' fruits and vegetables.

Fruit:	**Vegetable:**
huckleberry	Hass avocado
Color me BLUE	**Color me GREEN**
	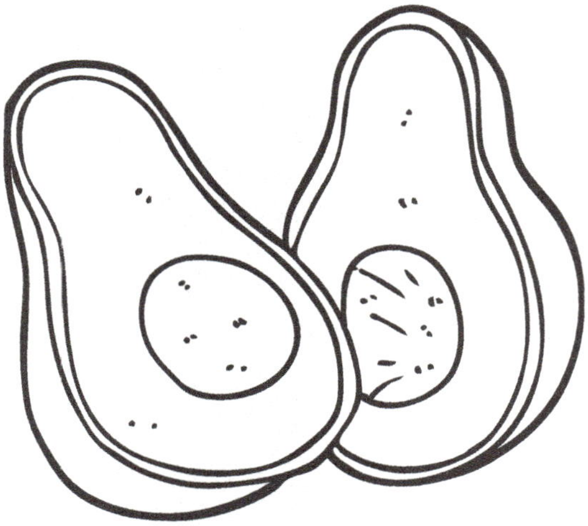

Trace & color me

GREEN

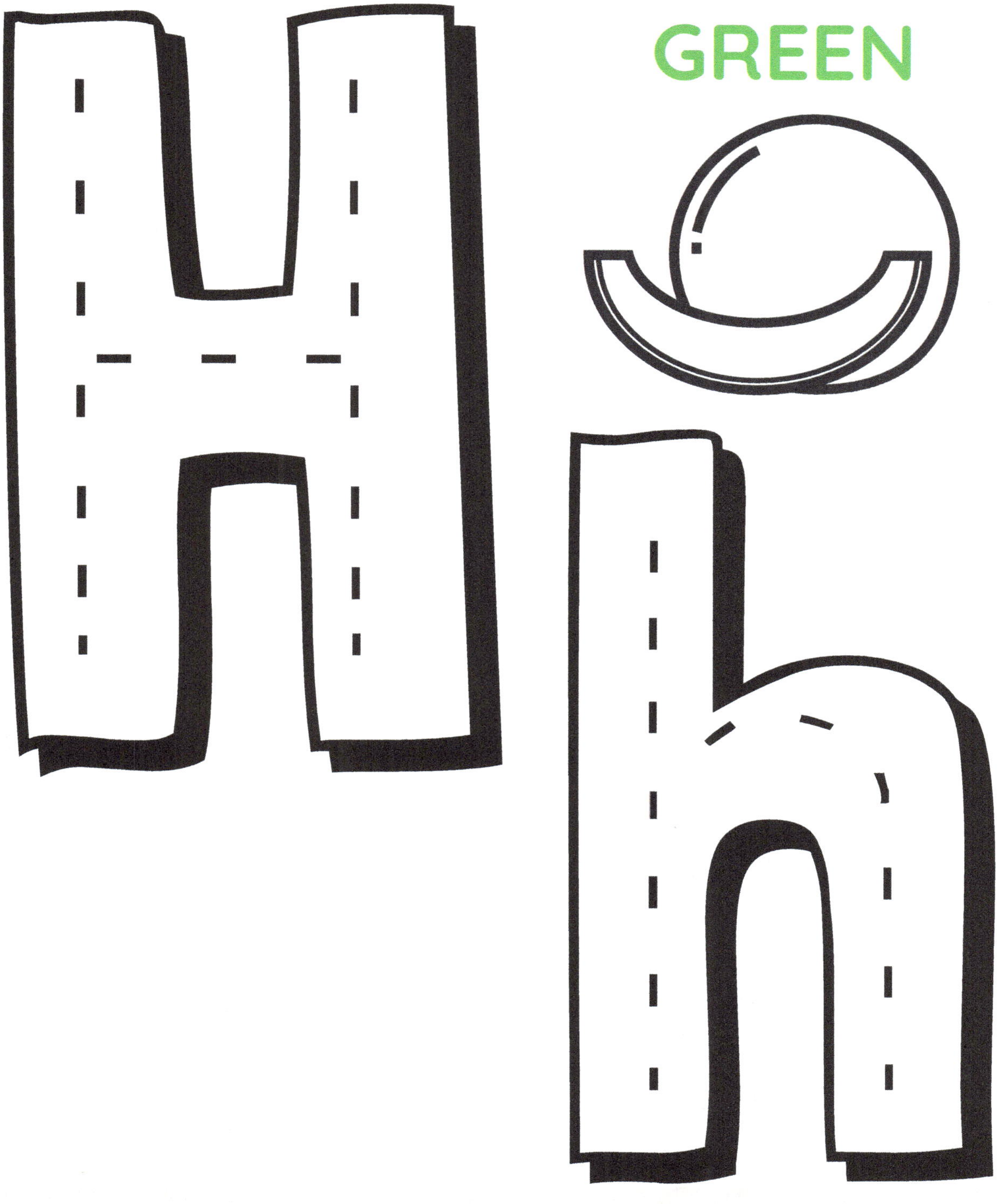

I

IDAHO POTATO

Fun Fact: Did you know that potatoes are 80% water and only 20% solid?

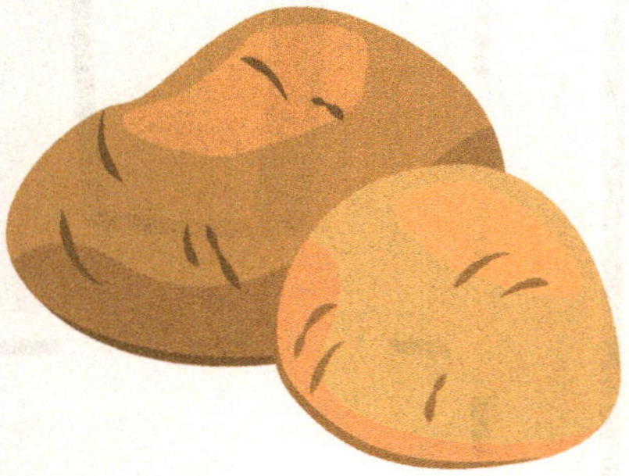

Directions: Color the 'i' fruits and vegetables.

Fruit: Indian prune	Vegetable: iceberg lettuce
Color me PURPLE	Color me GREEN
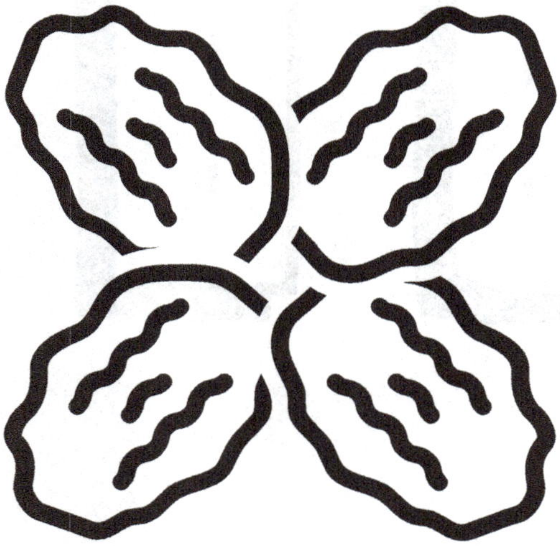	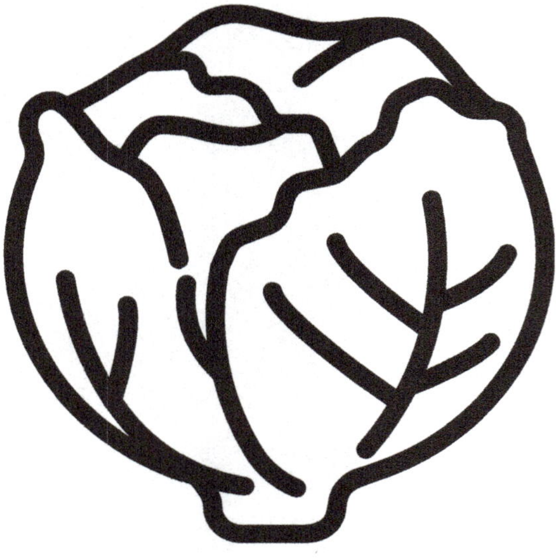

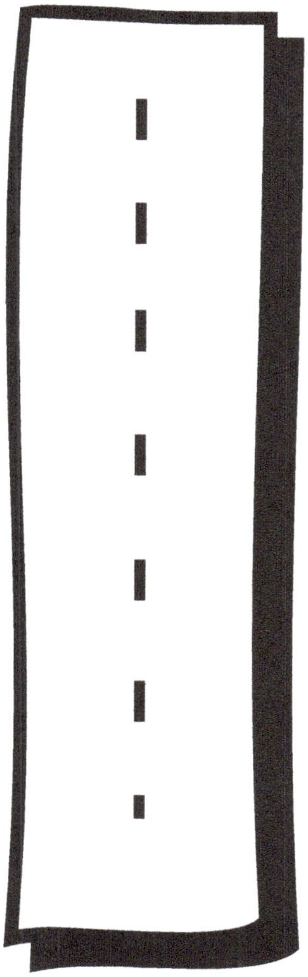

Trace & color me

BROWN

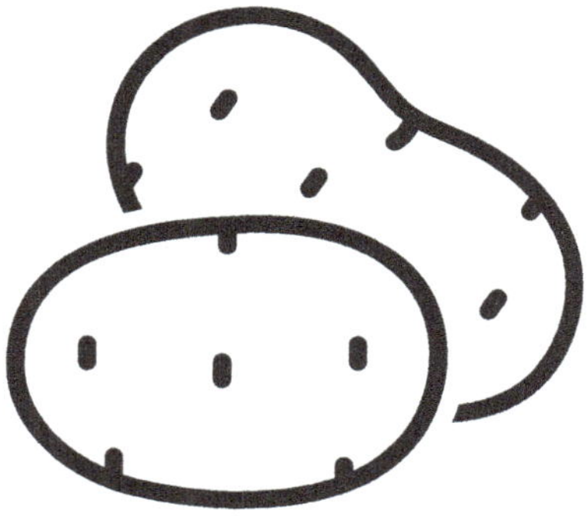

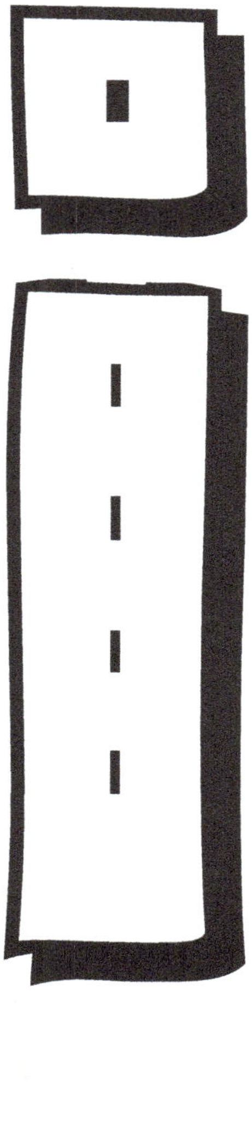

J

JICAMA

Crunchy like a chip,
eat with your
favorite dip!

Recipe in back of book!

Directions: Color the 'j' fruits and vegetables.

Fruit: jackfruit	**Vegetable:** jalapeño
Color me GREEN	**Color me GREEN**
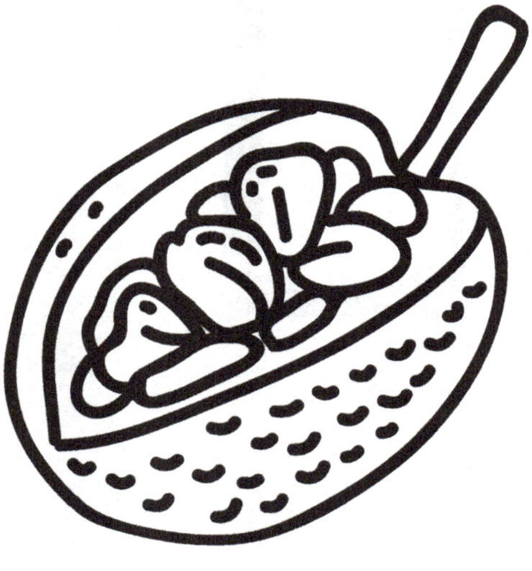	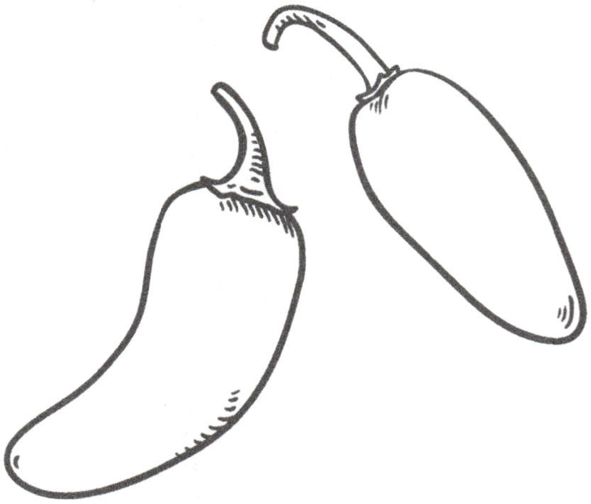

Trace & color me

BROWN

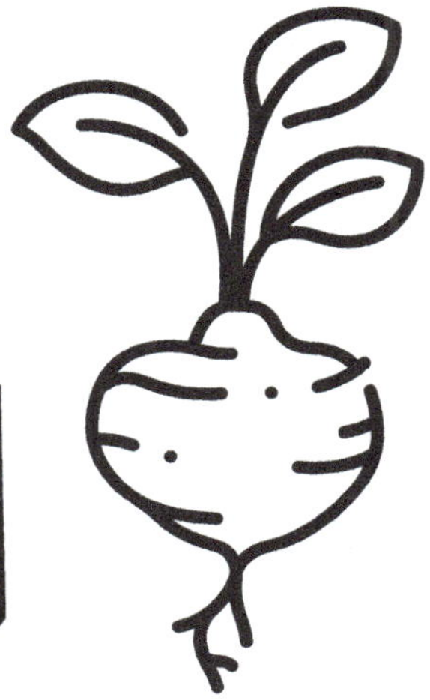

J j

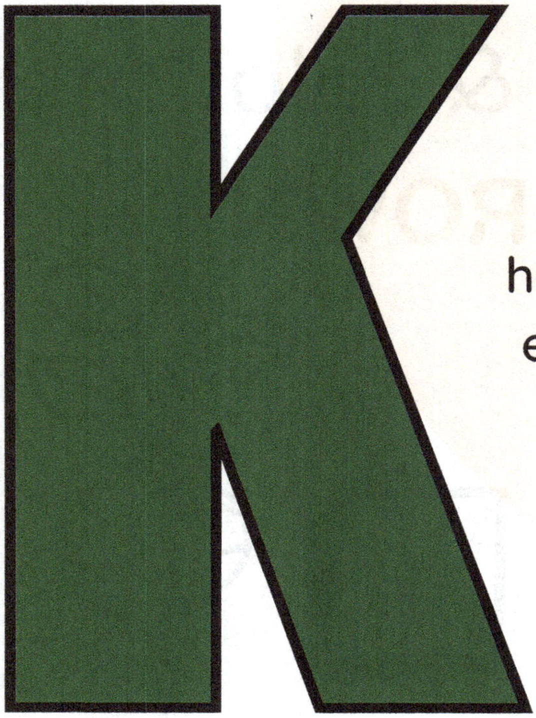

KALE

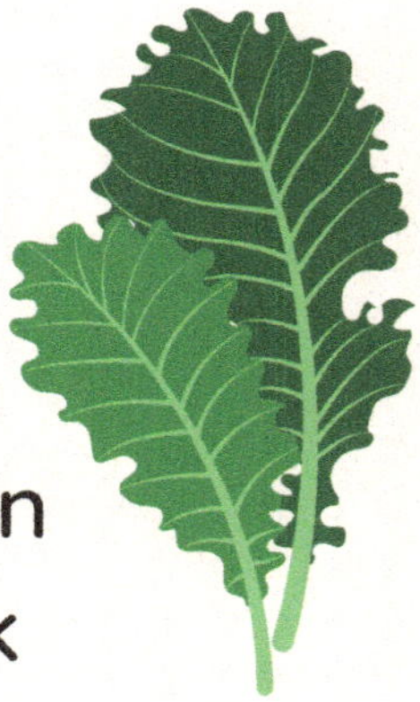

Kale is one of the healthiest lettuces you can eat along with other dark greens!

Recipe in back of book!

Directions: Color the 'k' fruits and vegetables.

Fruit: kiwi Color me GREEN 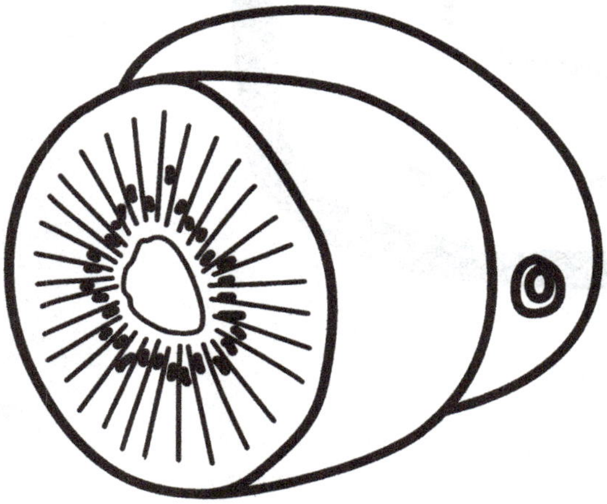	**Vegetable:** kohlrabi Color me PURPLE 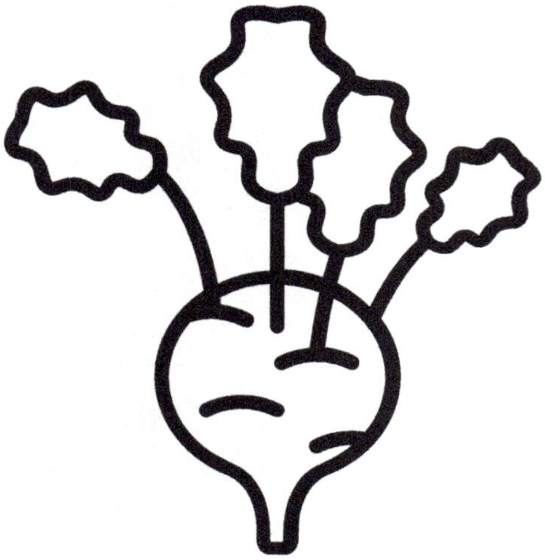

Trace & color me

GREEN

K k

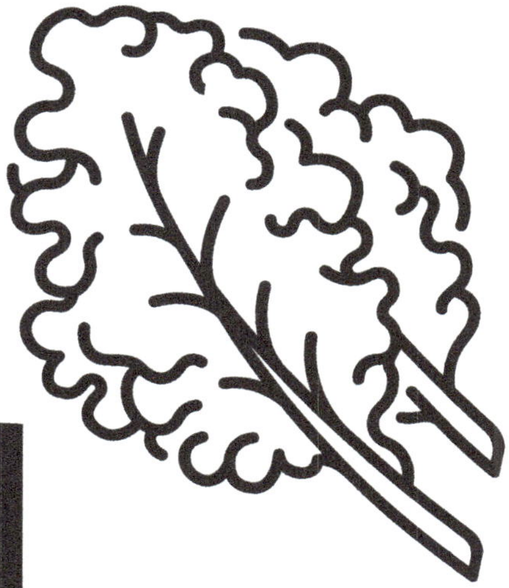

L

LEMON

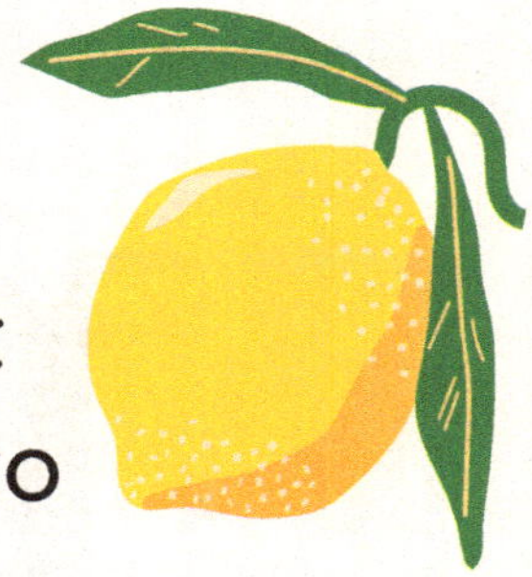

Lemons are a sour fruit that you can squeeze into your foods and drinks to add a citrusy flavor!

Directions: Color the 'l' fruits and vegetables.

Fruit:	Vegetable:
lime	lima bean
Color me GREEN	Color me GREEN
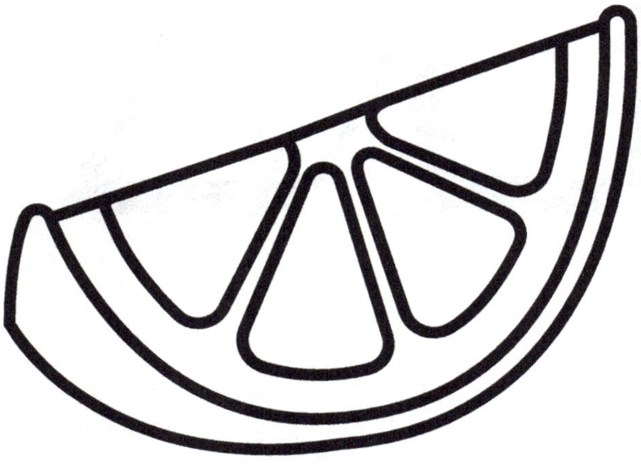	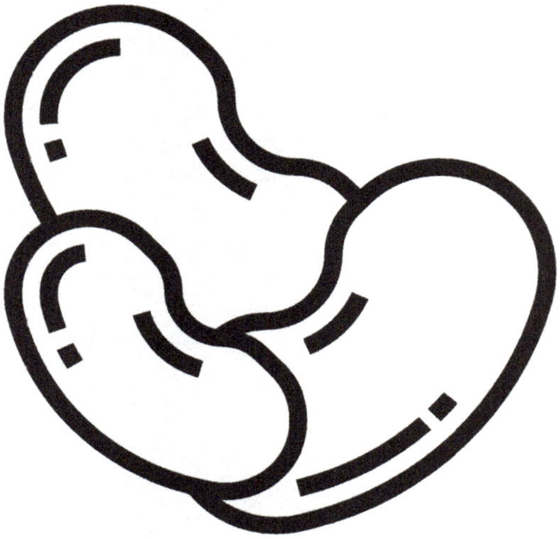

Trace & color me

YELLOW

M

MANGO

Eat this juicy fruit fresh or have it dried if you want a quick fruit snack to-go!

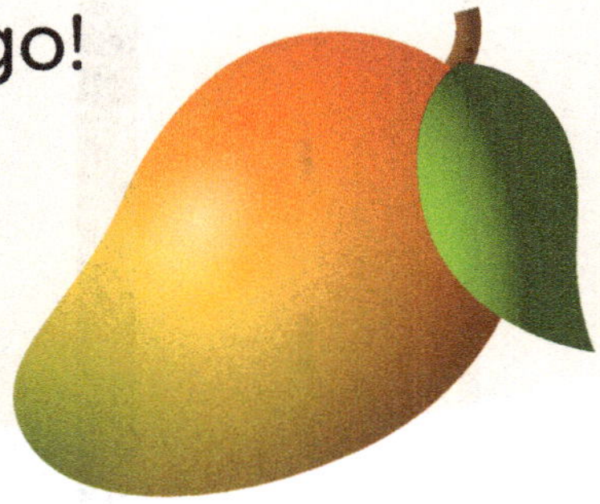

Directions: Color the 'm' fruits and vegetables.

Fruit: mandarin	**Vegetable:** mustard greens
Color me ORANGE	Color me GREEN
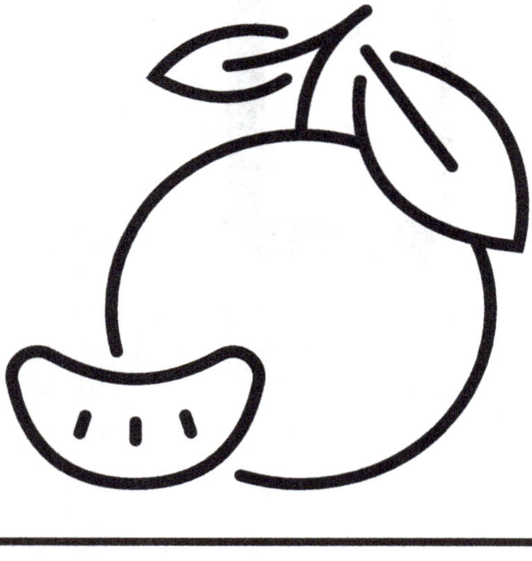	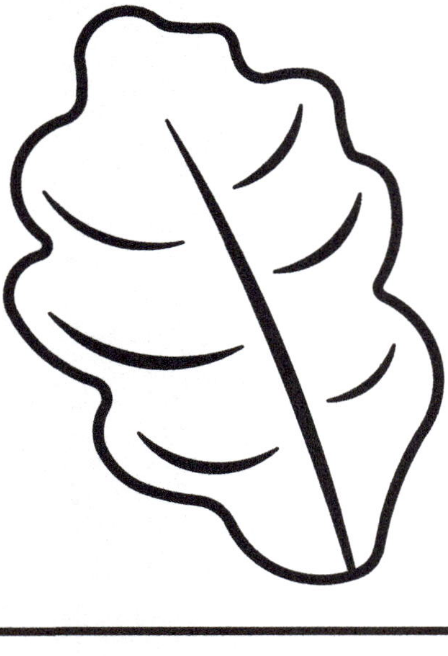

Trace & color me

ORANGE + RED

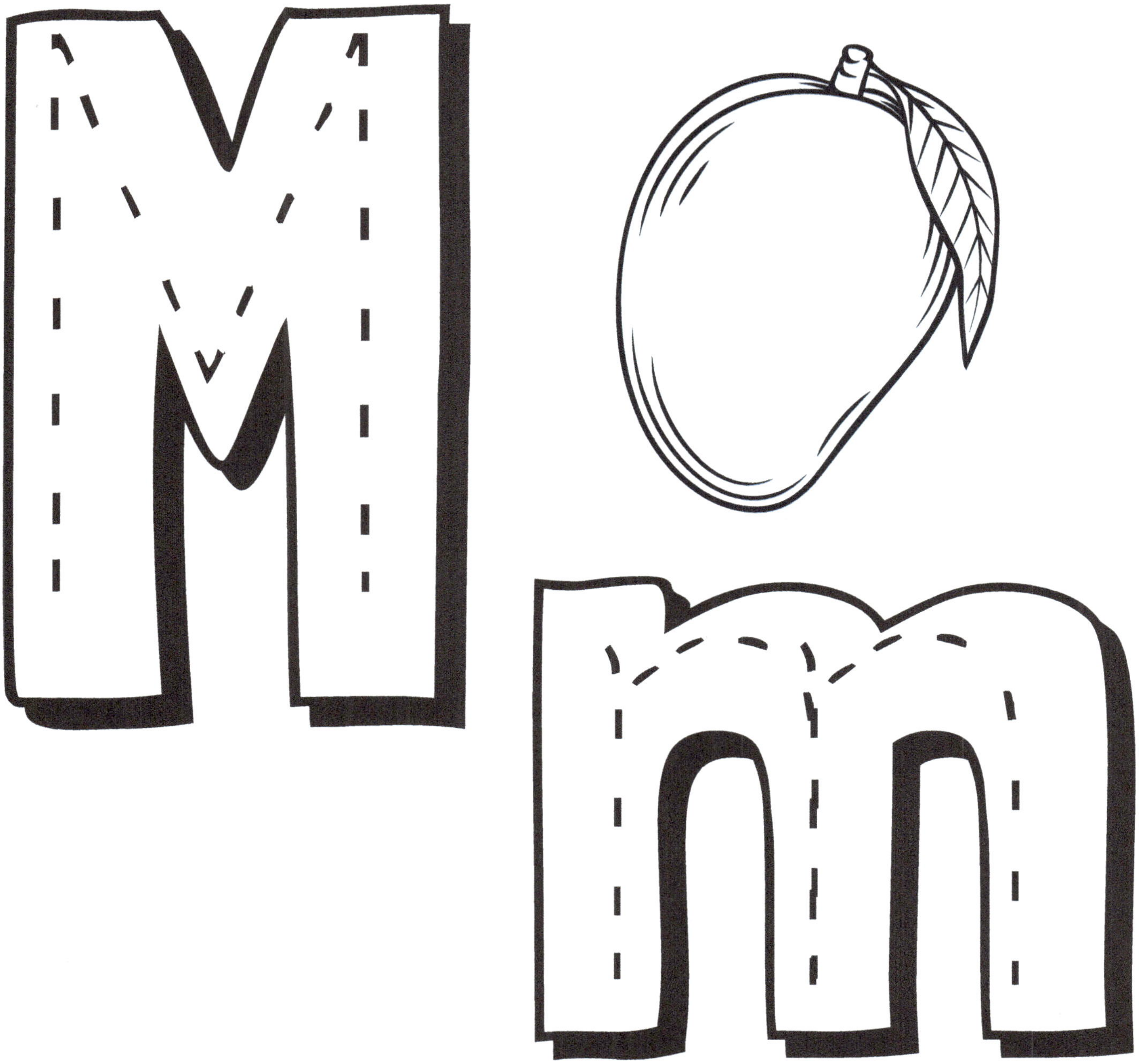

N

NECTARINE

These fruits are similar to peaches but unlike peaches, they don't have any fuzz!

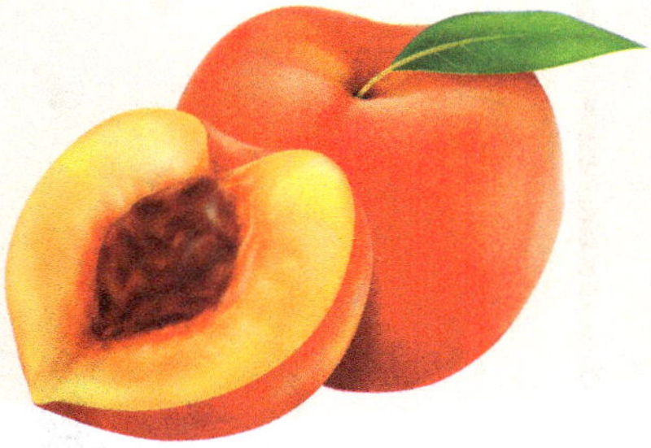

Directions: Color the 'n' fruits and vegetables.

Fruit:

Nashi pear

Color me YELLOW

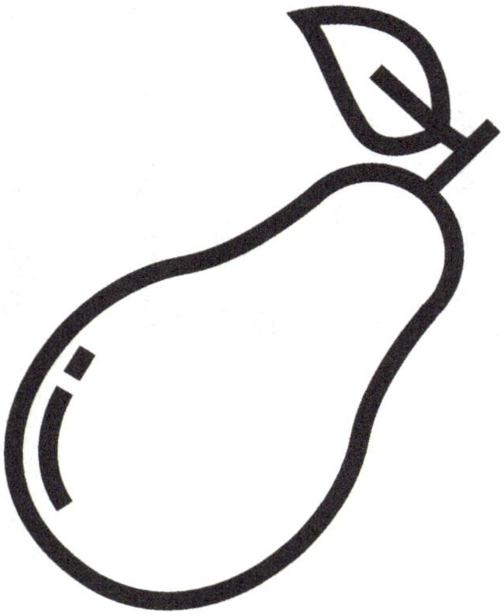

Vegetable:

navy bean

Color me WHITE

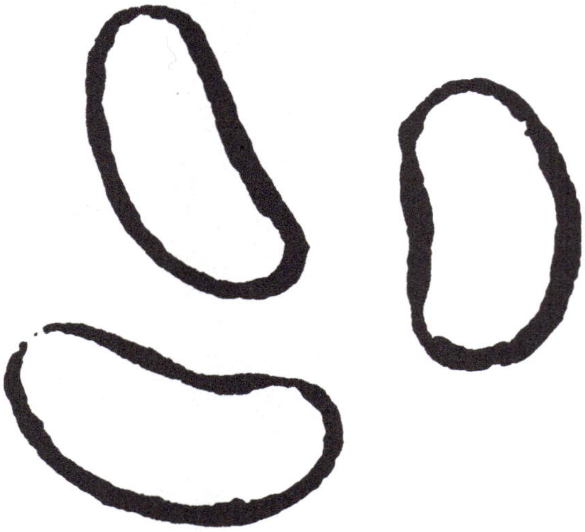

Trace & color me

ORANGE

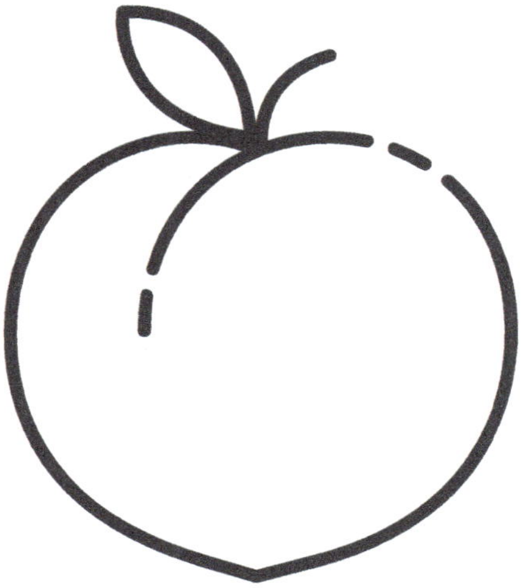

N

n

O

OLIVE

Eaten whole or in oil form, olives are rich in healthy fats that are very good for you!

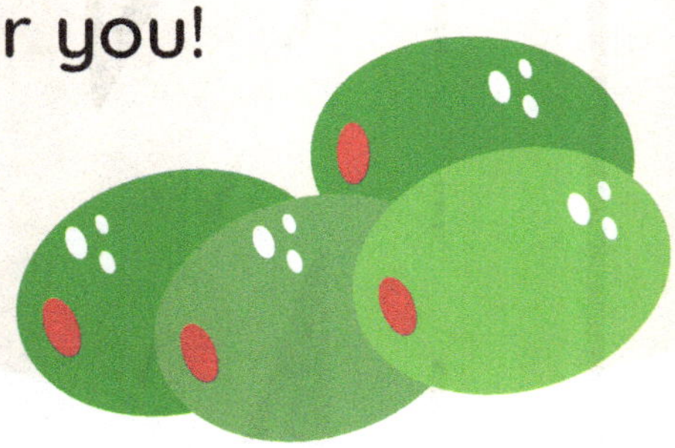

Directions: Color the 'o' fruits and vegetables.

Fruit:
orange

Color me ORANGE

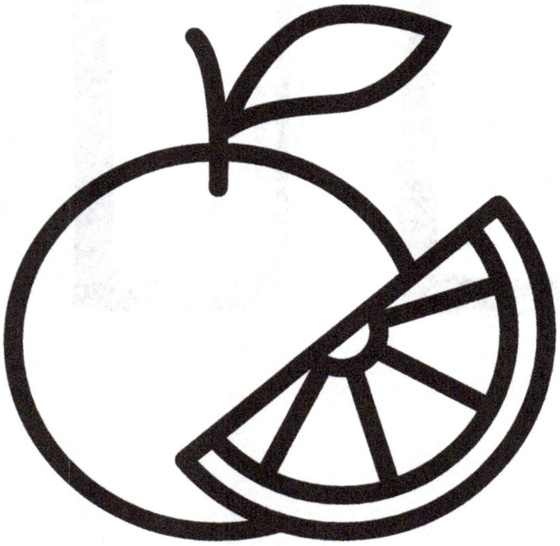

Vegetable:
okra

Color me GREEN

Trace & color me

GREEN

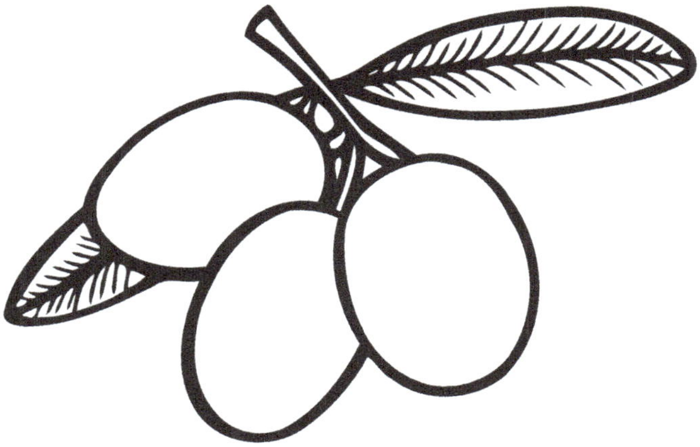

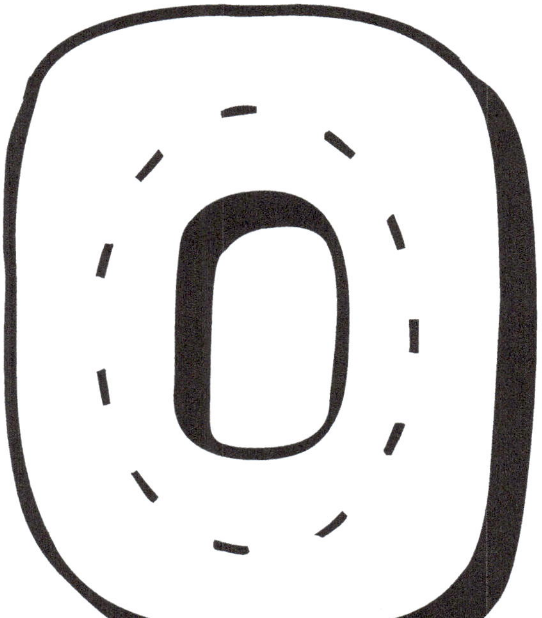

P

POMEGRANATE

Different than most fruits, you just eat the juicy seeds of the pomegranate!

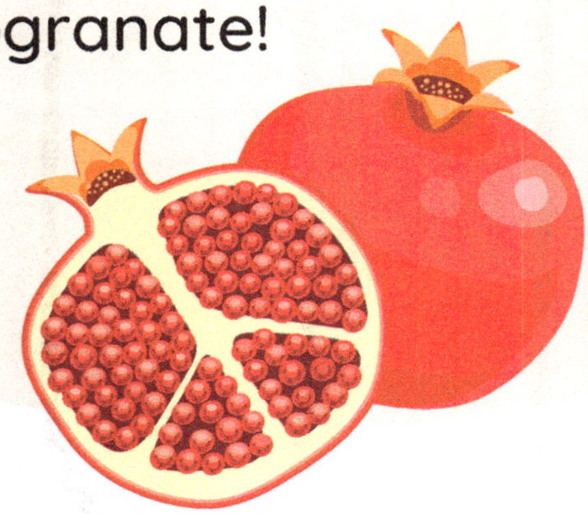

Directions: Color the 'p' fruits and vegetables.

Fruit: pineapple	**Vegetable:** pea
Color me YELLOW	**Color me GREEN**
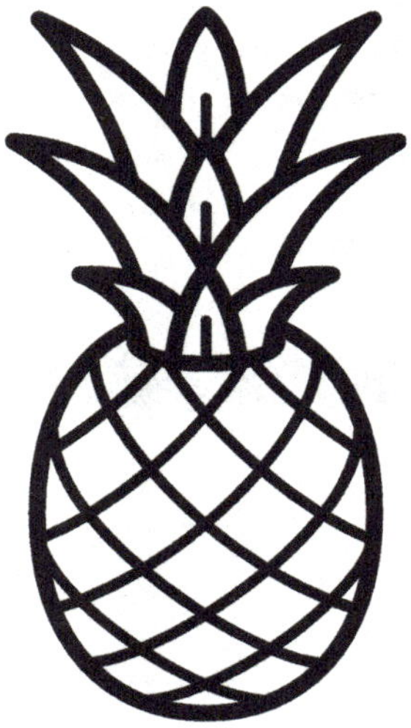	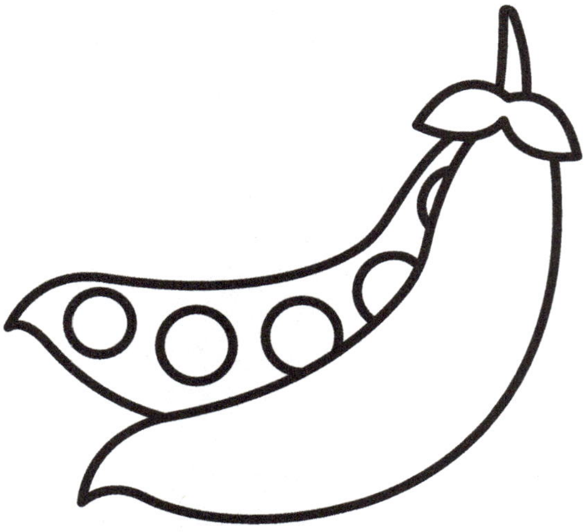

Trace & color me

RED

P

p

Q

QUINCE

Fun Fact: This pear-like fruit comes in all different shapes and is eaten cooked rather than raw!

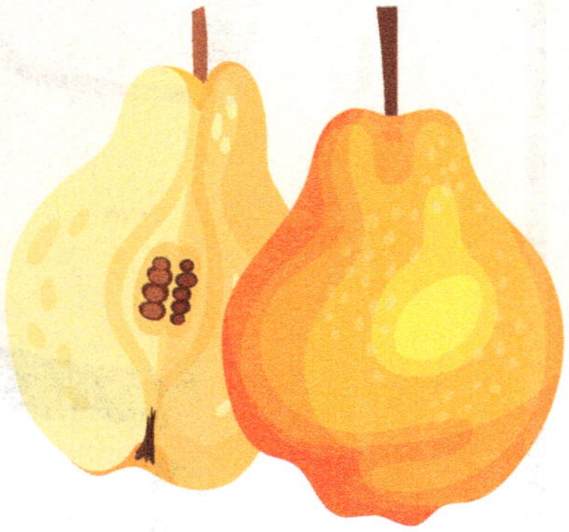

Directions: Color the 'q' fruits and vegetables.

Fruit:	Vegetable:
kumquat	squash
Color me ORANGE	Color me YELLOW
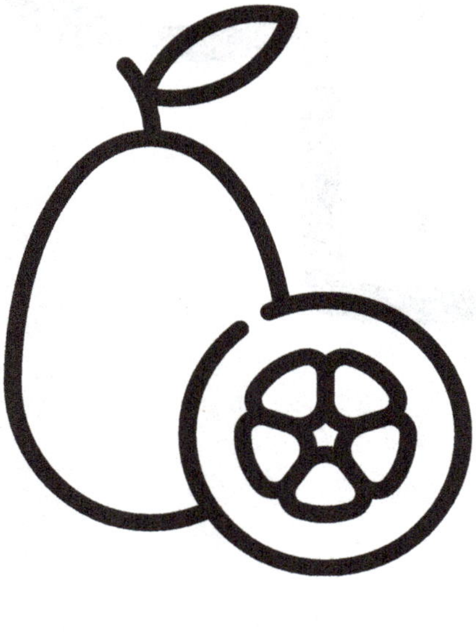	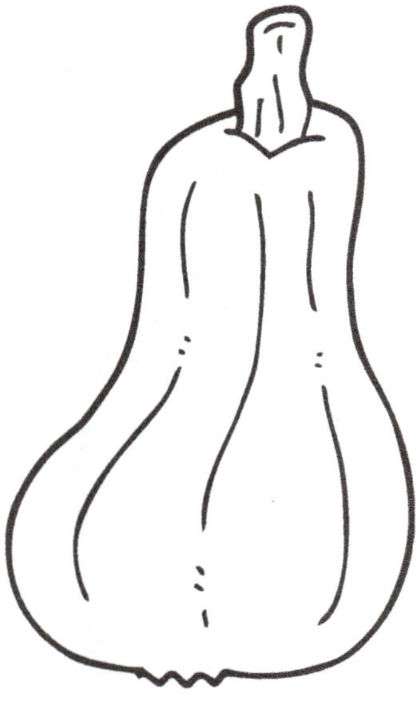

Trace & color me

YELLOW

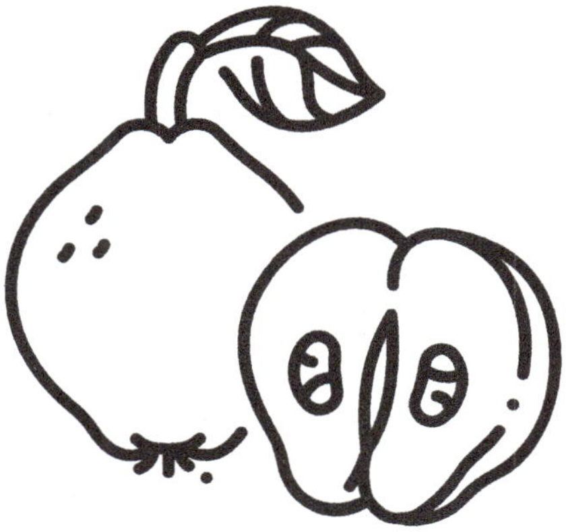

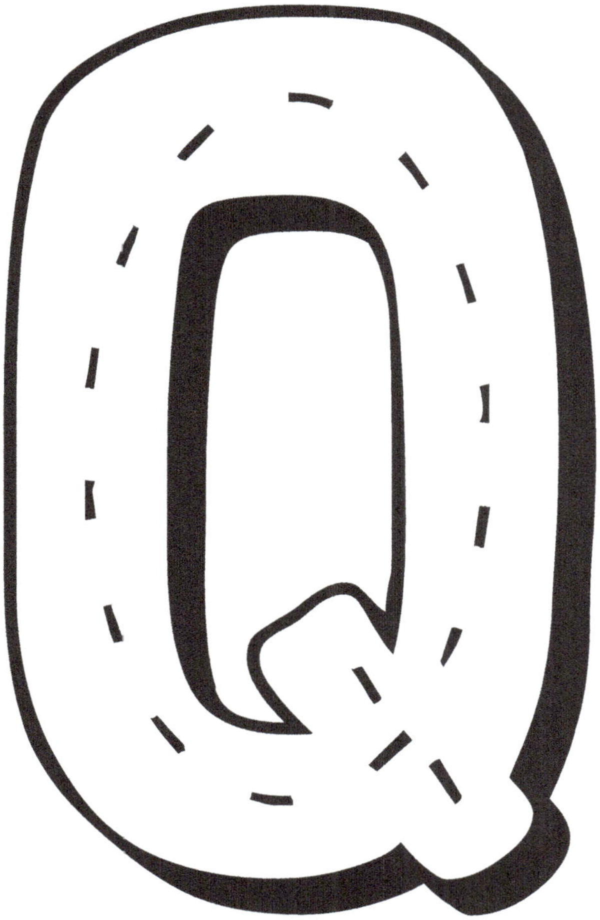

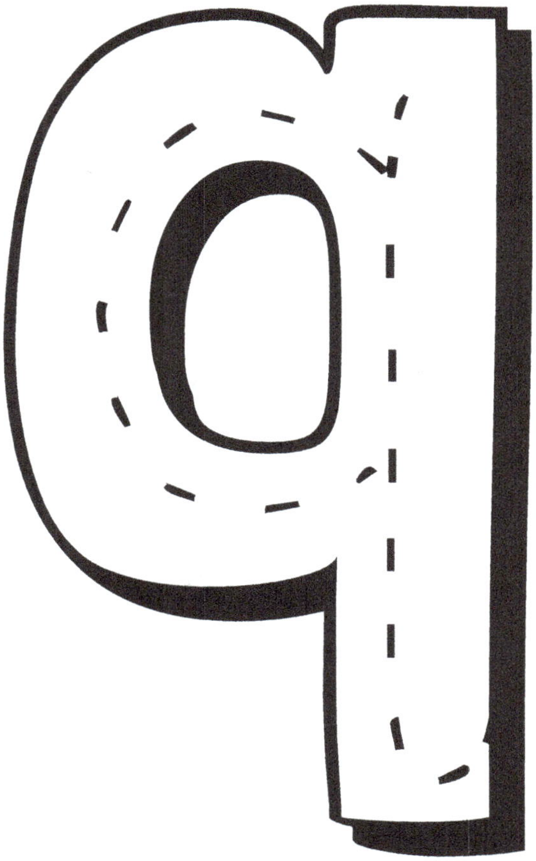

R

RADISH

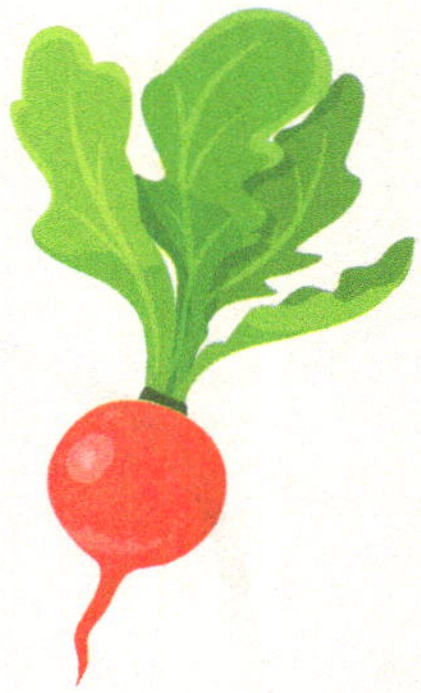

When eaten raw, this root vegetable is crunchy and tastes a bit spicy! Steam them for a more mild flavor.

Directions: Color the 'r' fruits and vegetables.

Fruit: raspberry	Vegetable: red cabbage
Color me RED	Color me PURPLE
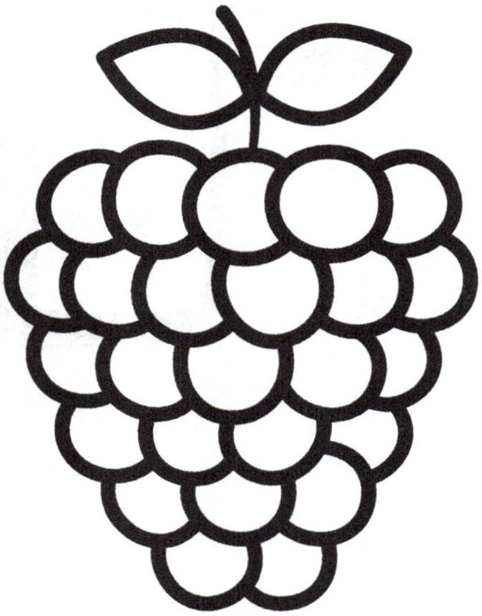	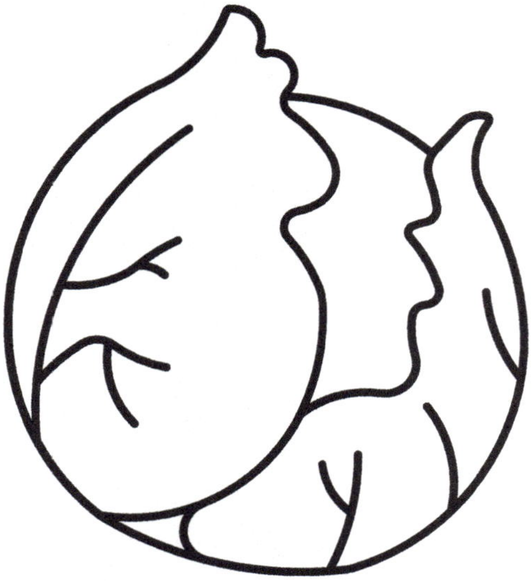

Trace & color me

RED

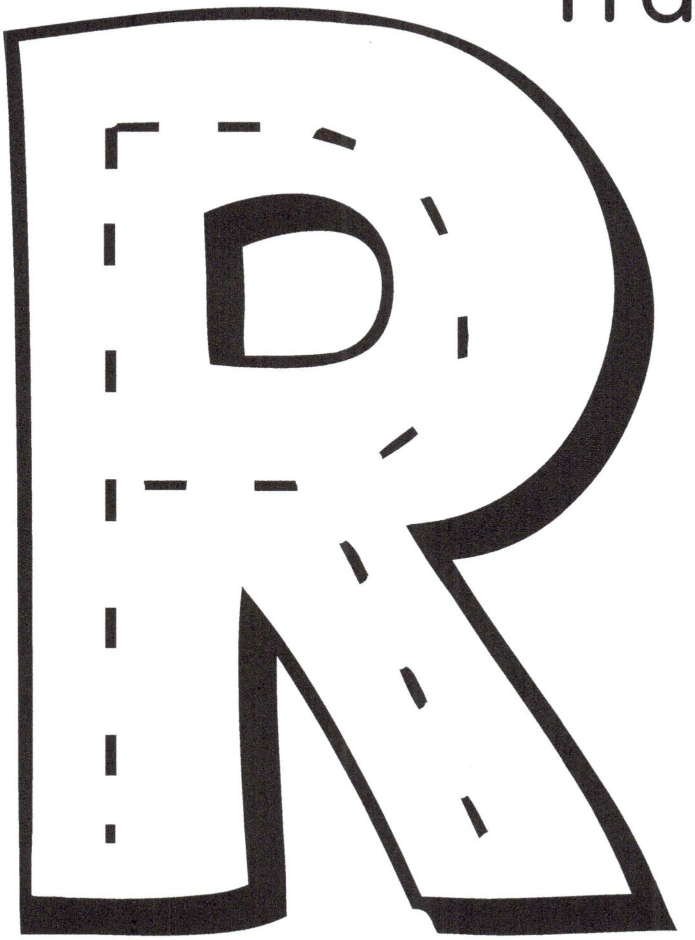

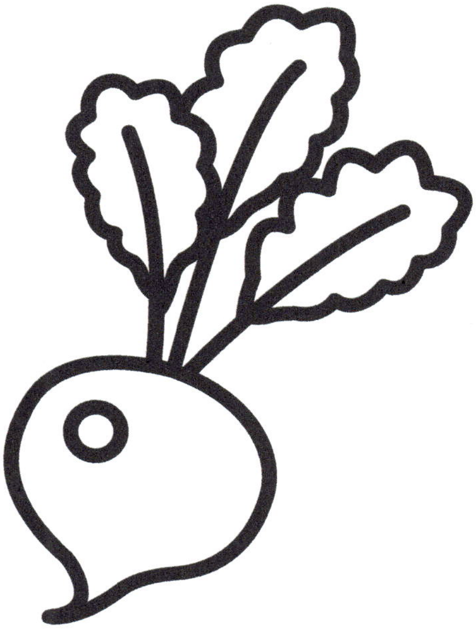

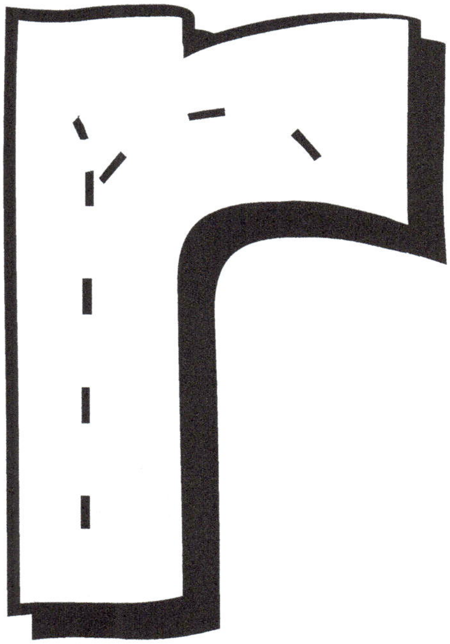

SPAGHETTI SQUASH

S

Once cooked, this squash looks like spaghetti noodles! Eat them as you would eat noodles with your favorite sauce.

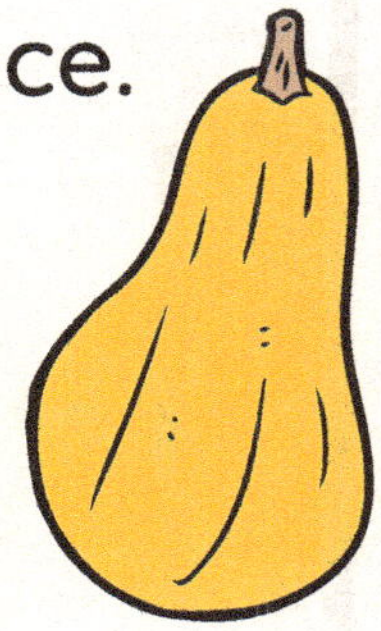

Recipe in back of book!

Directions: Color the 's' fruits and vegetables.

Fruit: strawberry	Vegetable: spinach
Color me RED	Color me GREEN
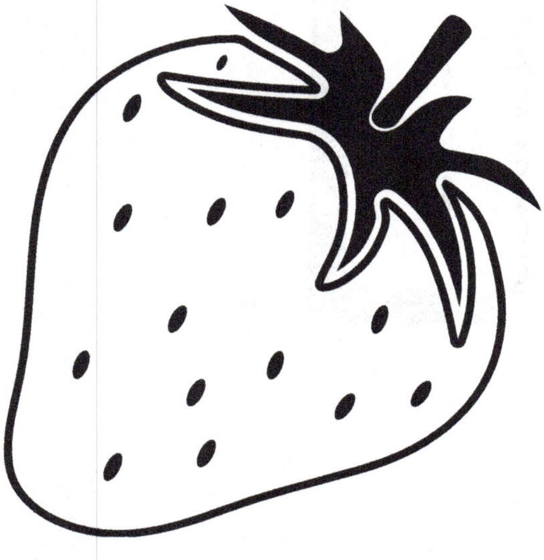	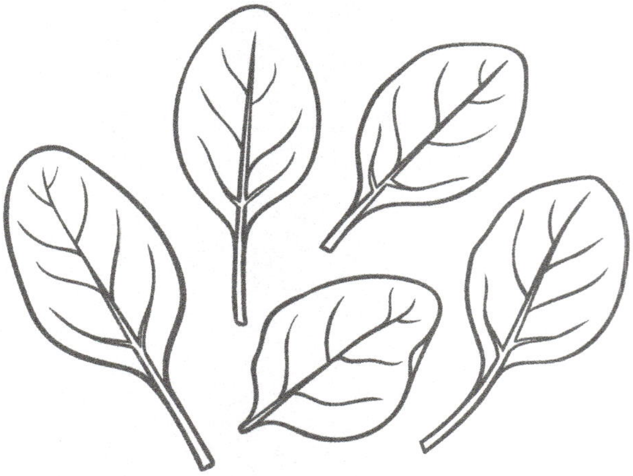

Trace & color me

YELLOW

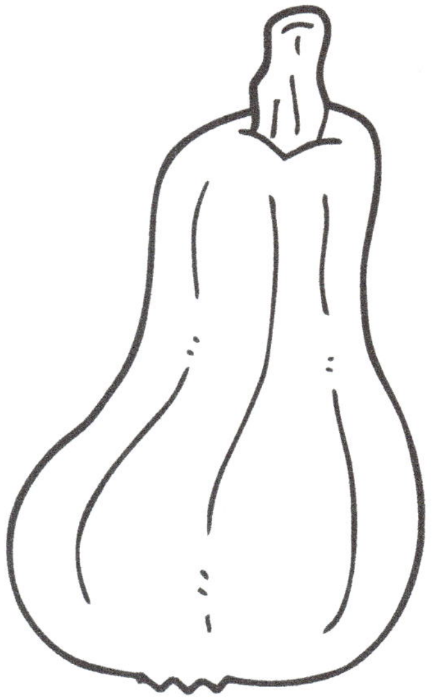

S s

T

TOMATO

Fun Fact: Tomatoes aren't always red— they can be yellow, green, pink, orange, or even black!

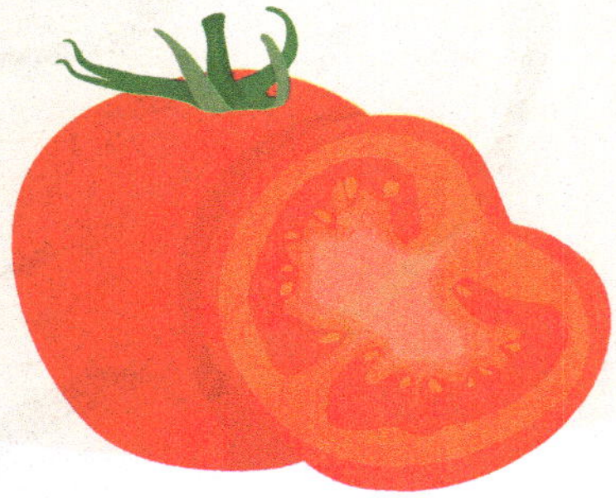

Directions: Color the 't' fruits and vegetables.

Fruit: tangerine	Vegetable: turnip
Color me ORANGE	Color me PURPLE
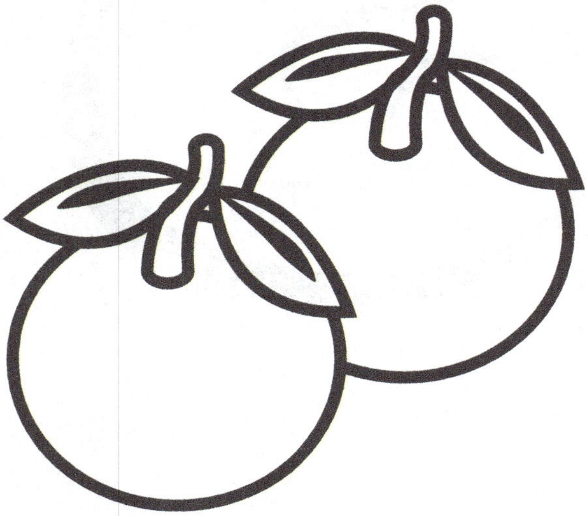	

Trace & color me

RED

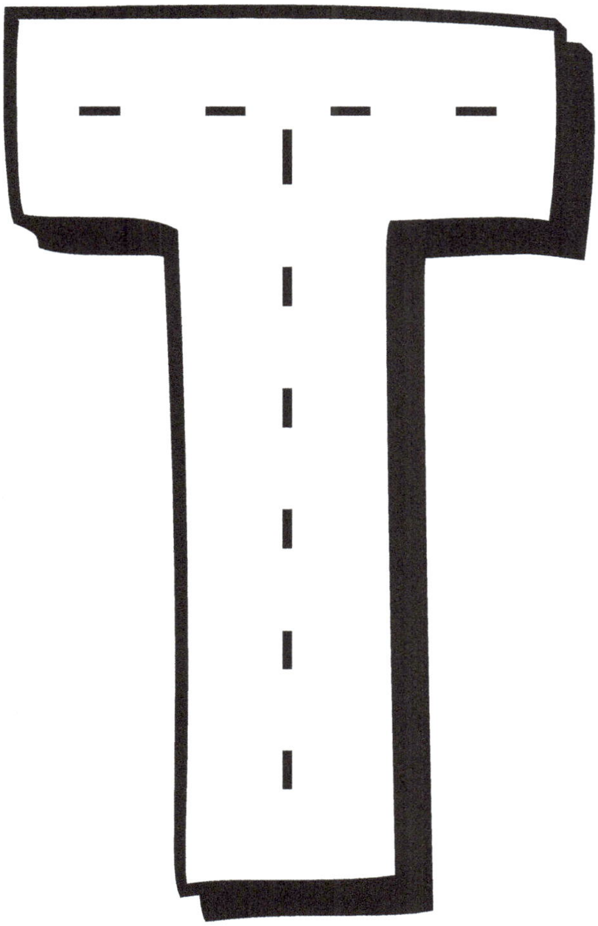

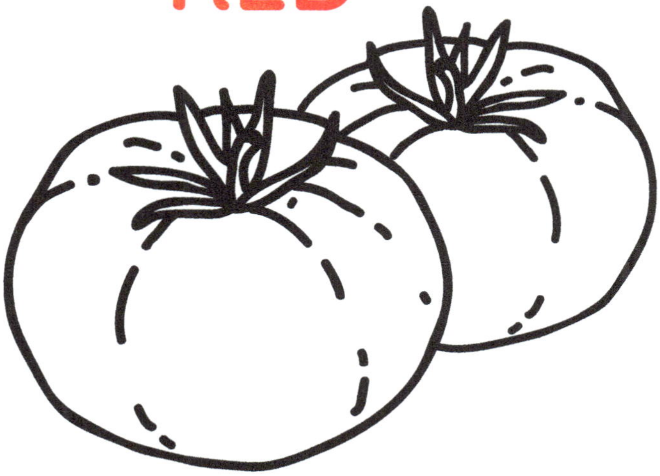

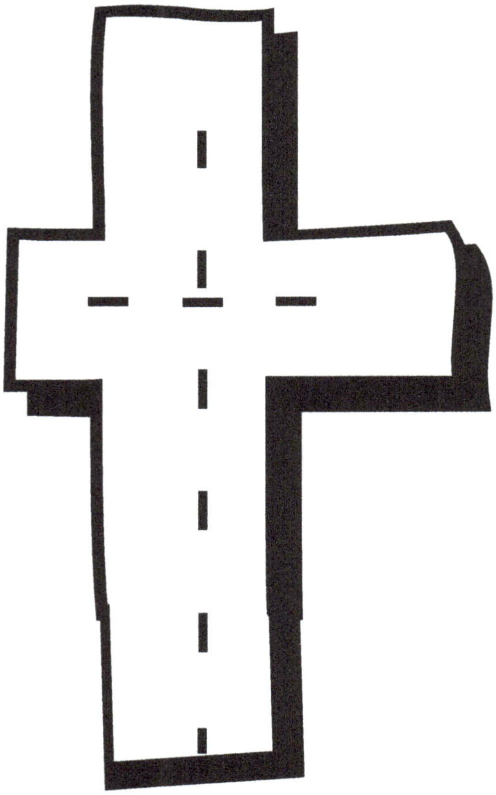

UMBRELLA SQUASH

U

Fun Fact: Umbrella squash is a nickname for pattypan squash because— you guessed it— it looks like an umbrella!

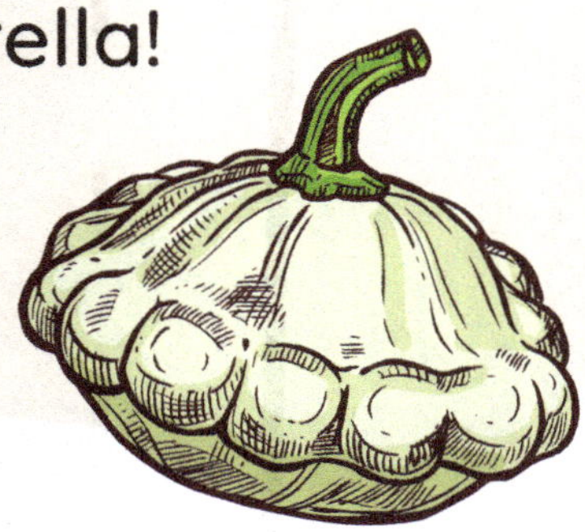

Directions: Color the 'u' fruits and vegetables.

Fruit:	**Vegetable:**
ugli (Jamaican tangelo)	ube (sweet potato)
Color me ORANGE	Color me PURPLE
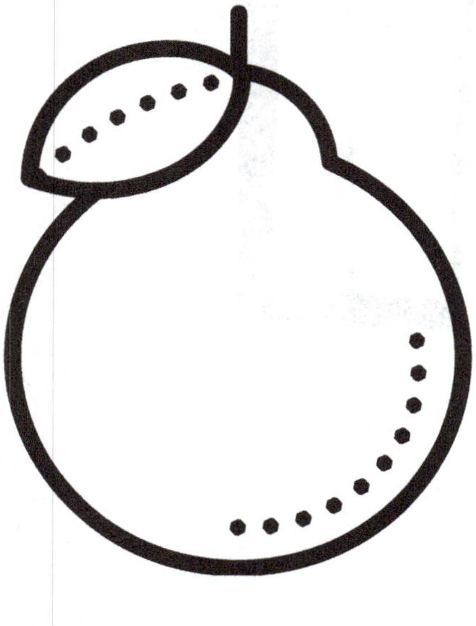	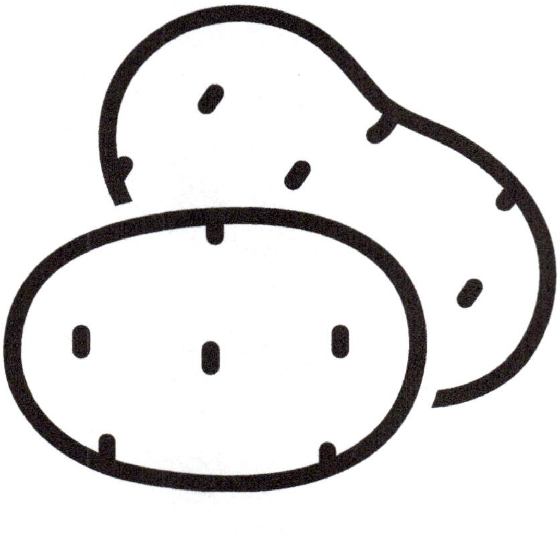

Trace & color me

YELLOW

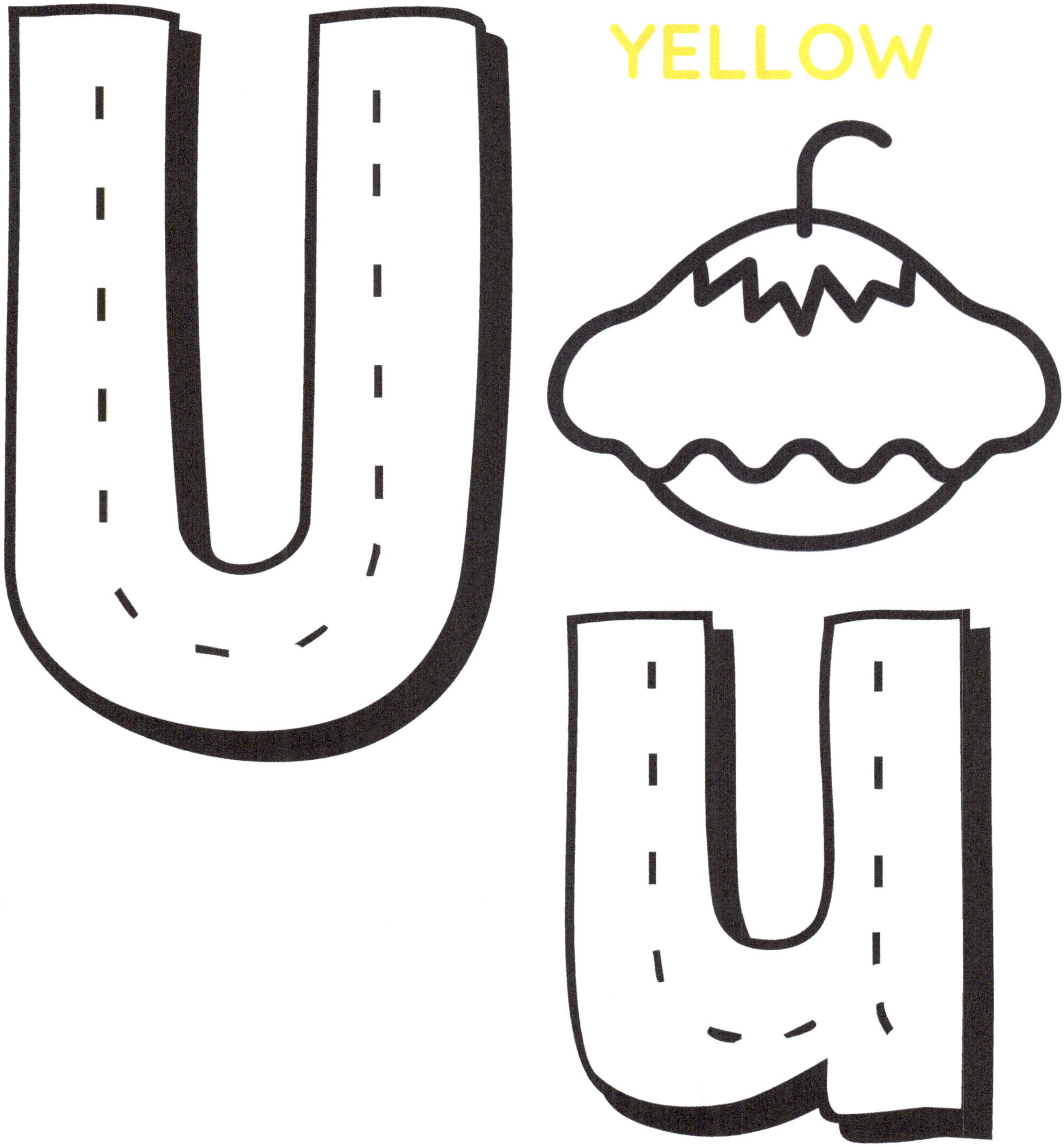

VALENCIA ORANGE

V

These juicy fruits are loaded with vitamin C which helps to keep you healthy and your immune system strong!

Recipe in back of book!

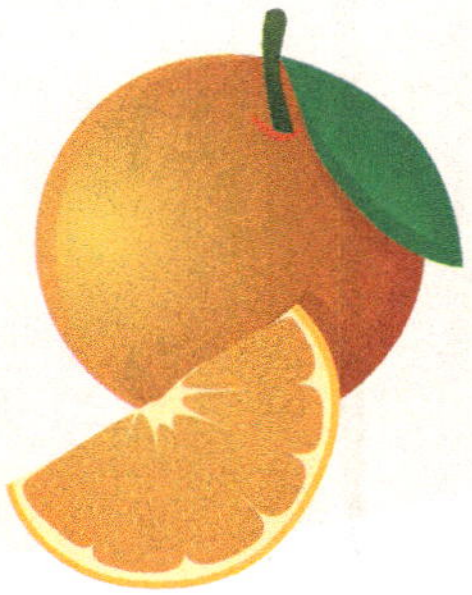

Directions: Color the 'v' fruits and vegetables.

Fruit: vine grapes	**Vegetable:** Vidalia onion
Color me PURPLE	Color me YELLOW
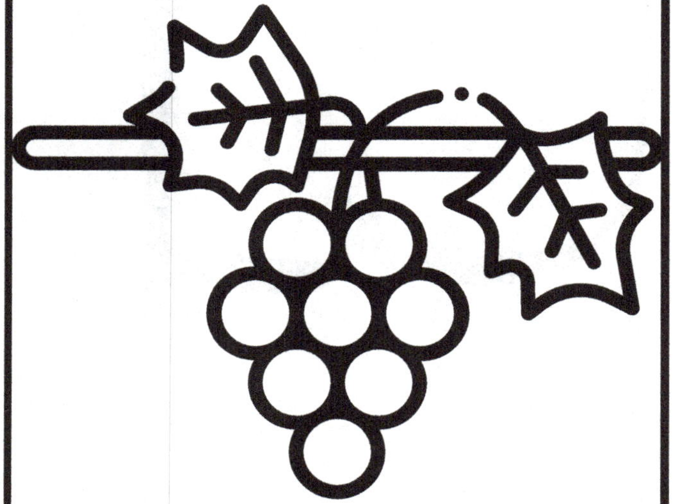	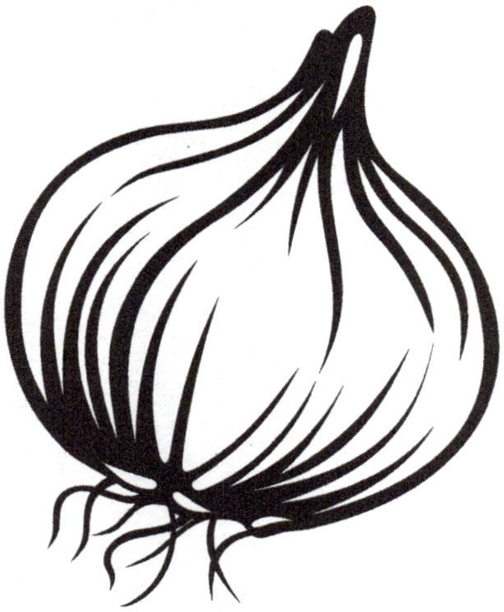

Trace & color me

ORANGE

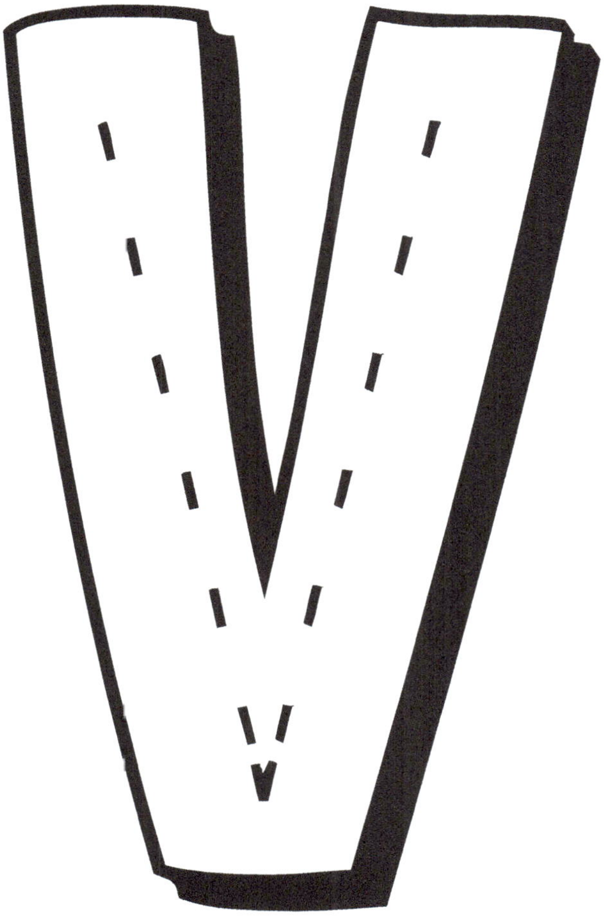

WATERMELON

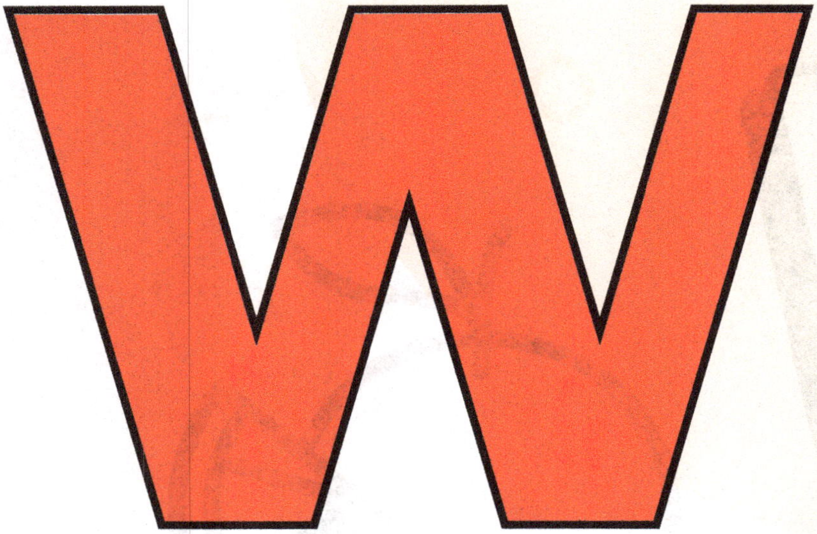

Fun Fact: The largest watermelon ever grown was from Arkansas in 2005 and it weighed 268 pounds!

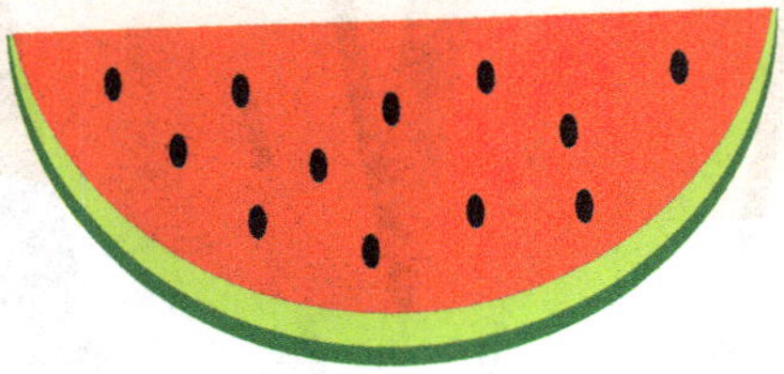

Directions: Color the 'w' fruits and vegetables.

Fruit: white peach	Vegetable: white carrot
Color me ORANGE	Color me WHITE
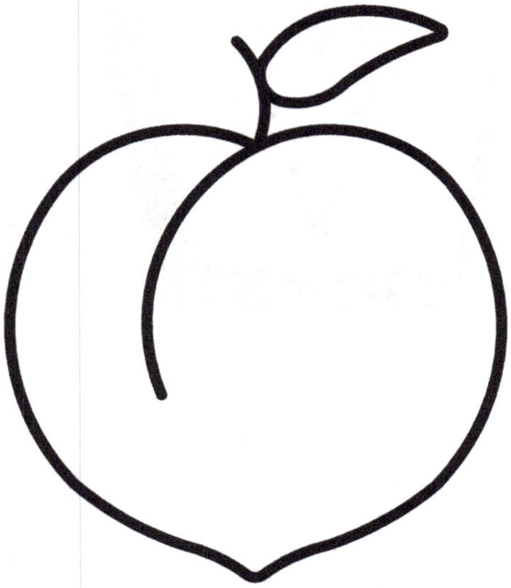	

Trace & color me

GREEN + RED

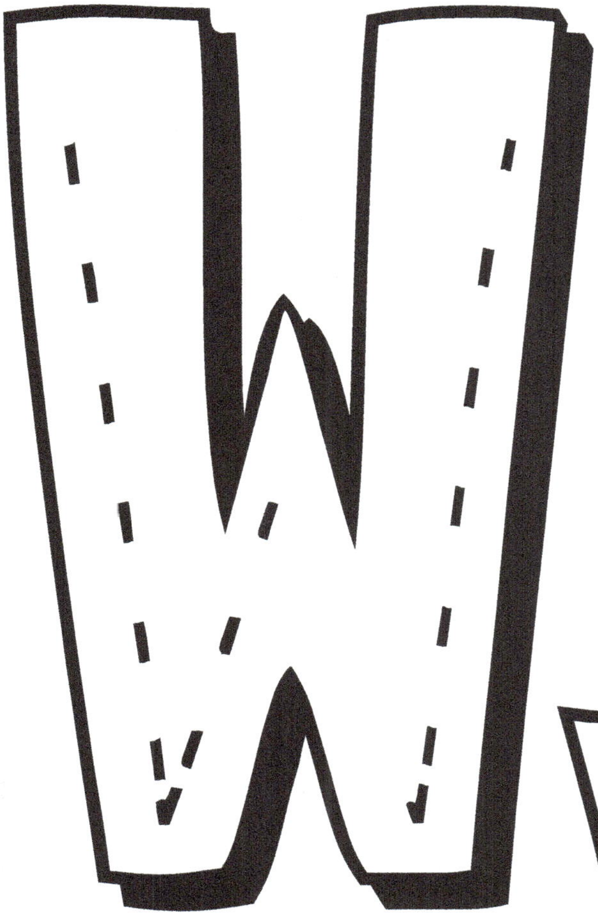

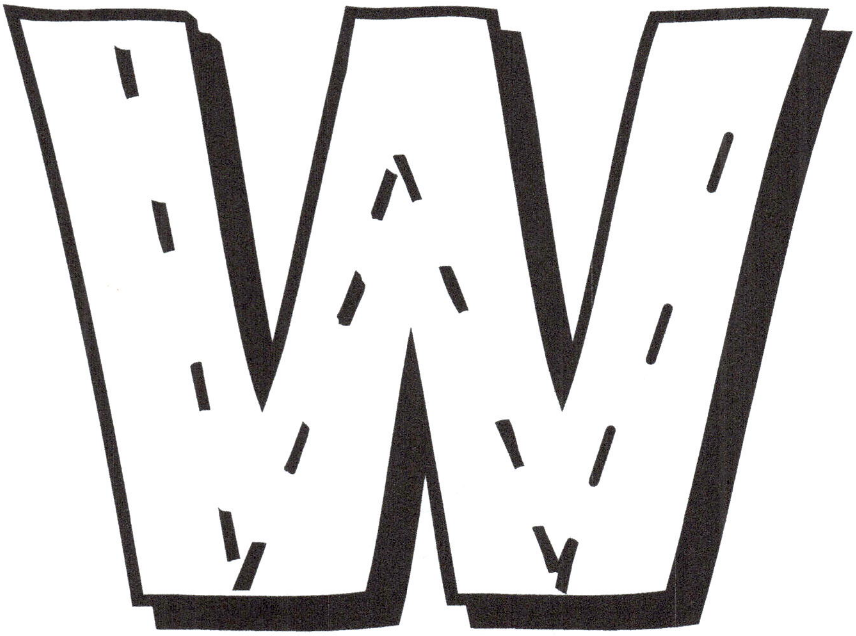

X

XIMENIA

This South African fruit has many nicknames like monkey plum and hog plum. They are only found in the wild!

Directions: Color the 'x' fruits and vegetables.

Fruit:	**Vegetable:**
xigua (African watermelon)	wax bean
Color me RED	**Color me GREEN**
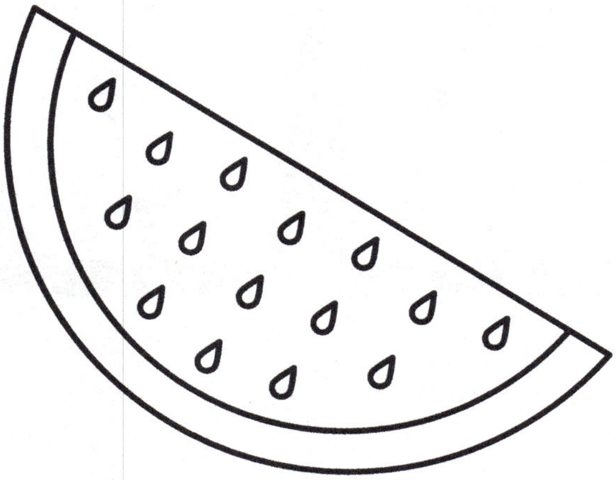	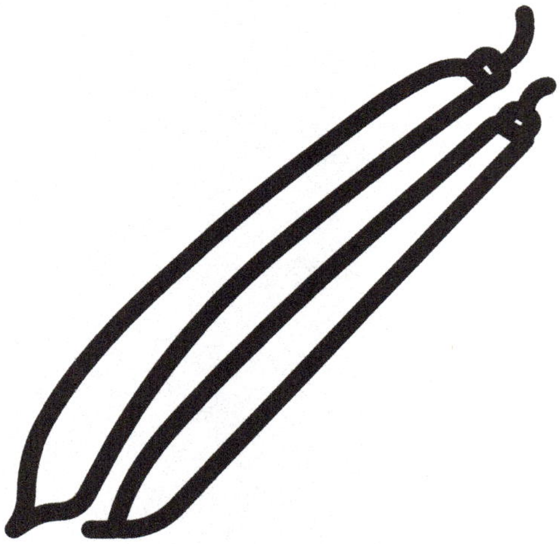

Trace & color me

YELLOW

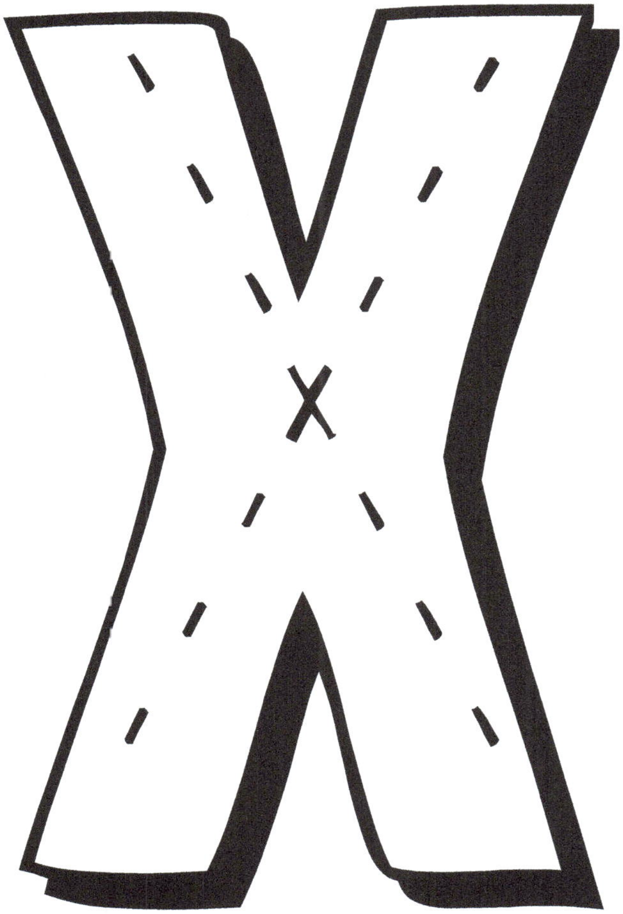

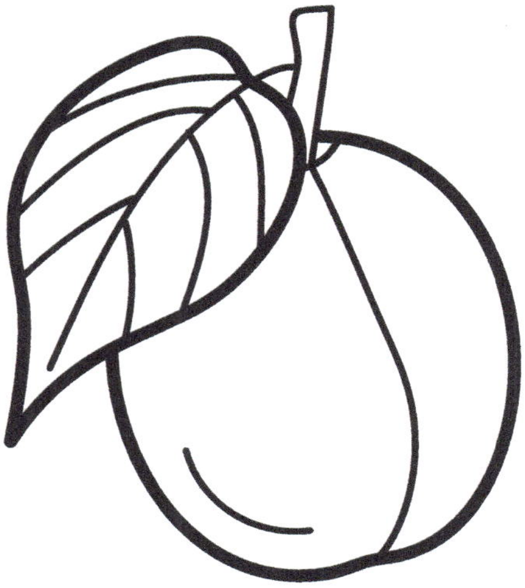

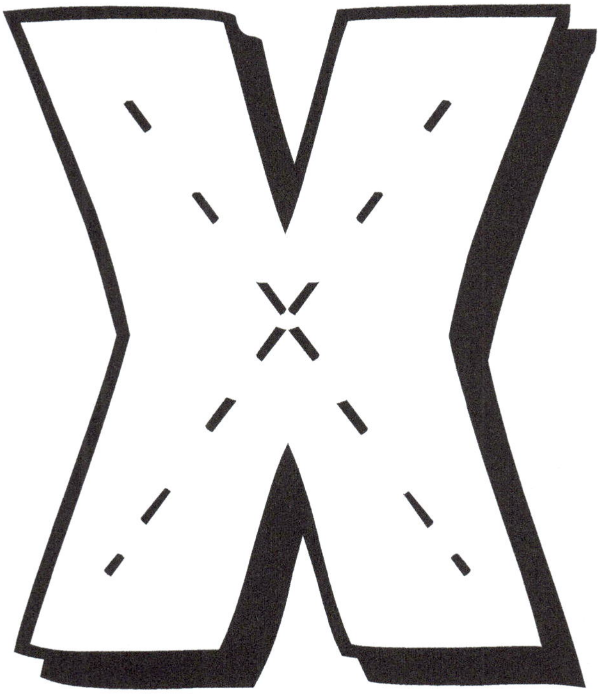

Y

YAM

Yams are a type of sweet potato and can vary in all different shapes and sizes—even up to 100 pounds!

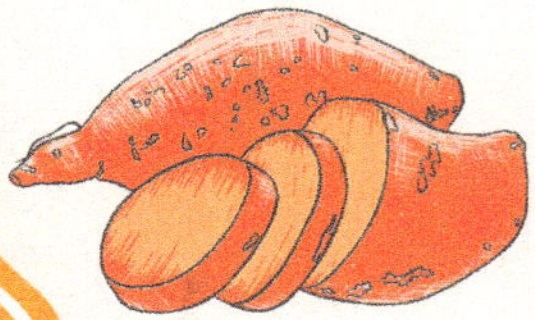

Recipe in back of book!

Directions: Color the 'y' fruits and vegetables.

Fruit:	Vegetable:
yellow plum	yellow bell pepper
Color me YELLOW	Color me YELLOW
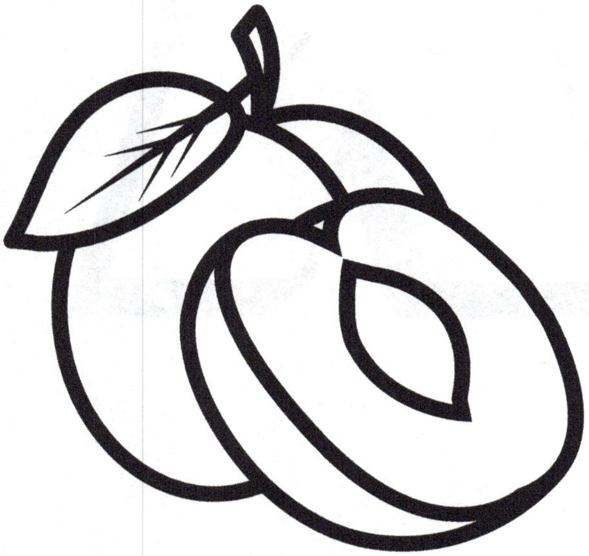	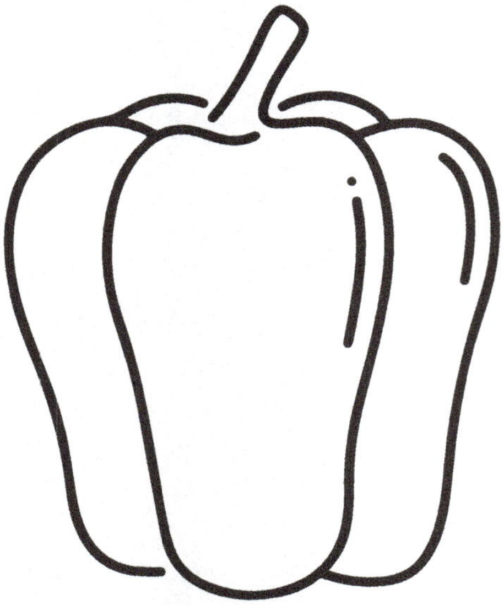

Trace & color me

ORANGE

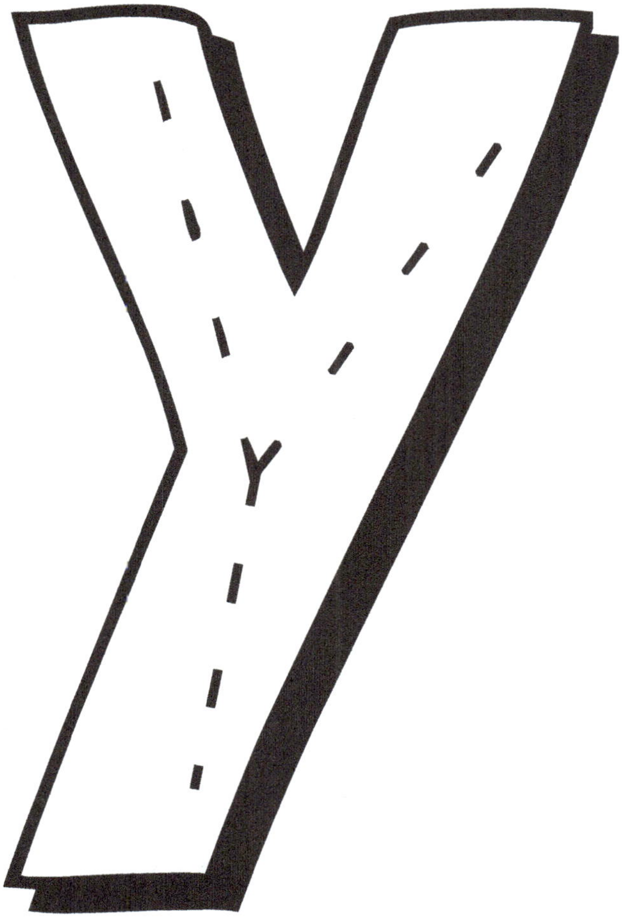

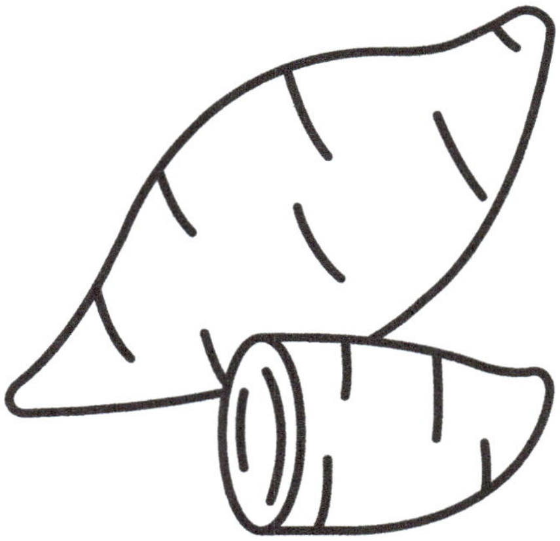

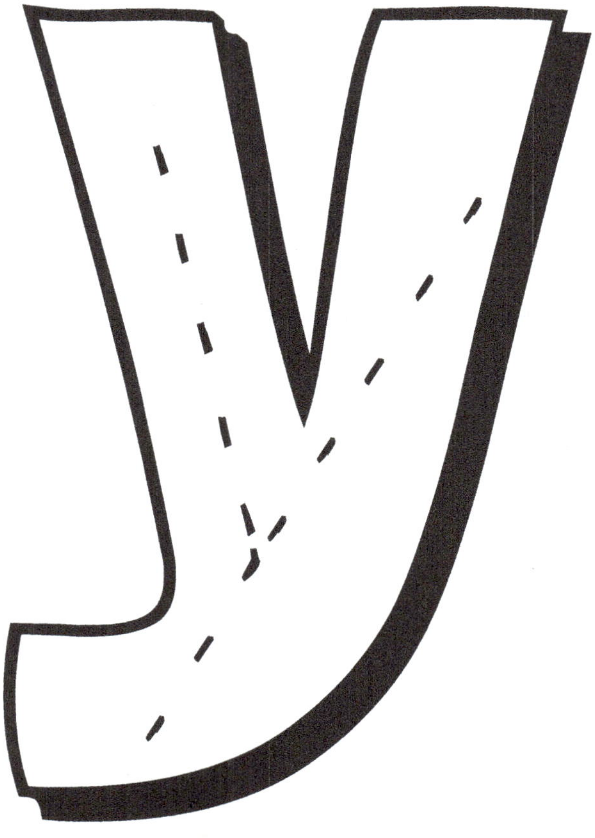

Z

ZUCCHINI

This vegetable is very versatile as it can be eaten in many different ways: raw, sautéed, noodles, soups, and even baked goods!

Recipe in back of book!

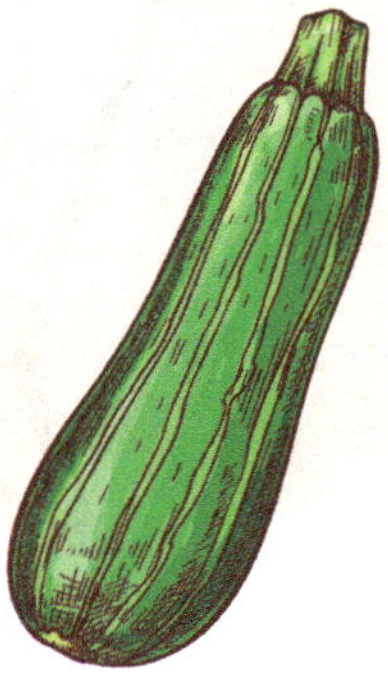

Directions: Color the 'z' fruits and vegetables.

Fruit: zesty lemon Color me YELLOW	Vegetable: fuzzy squash Color me GREEN
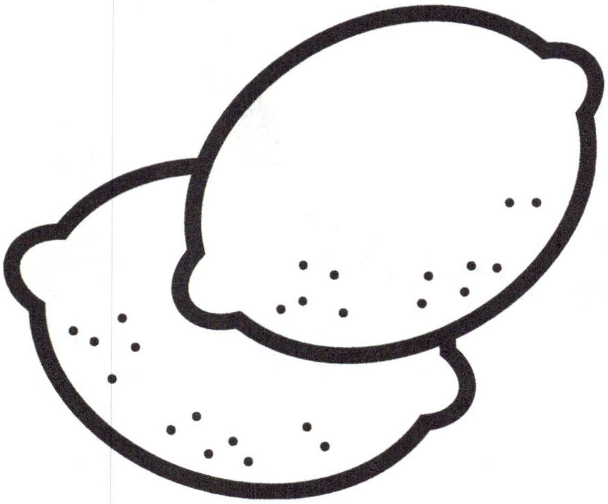	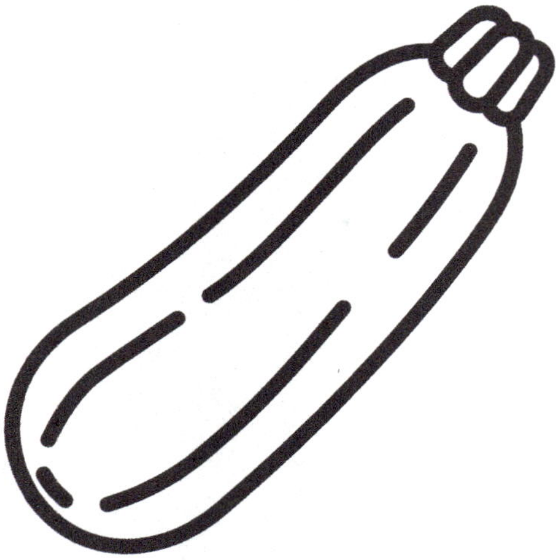

Trace & color me

GREEN

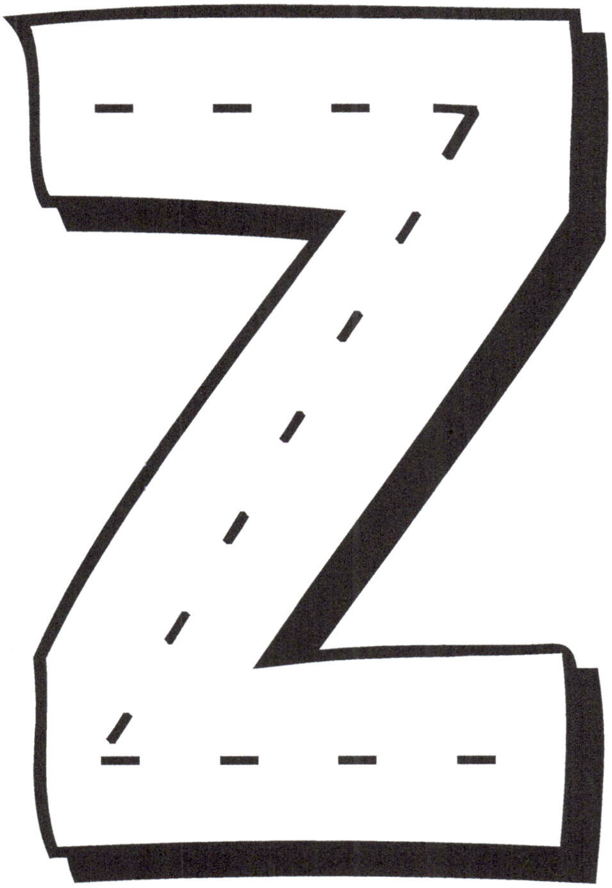

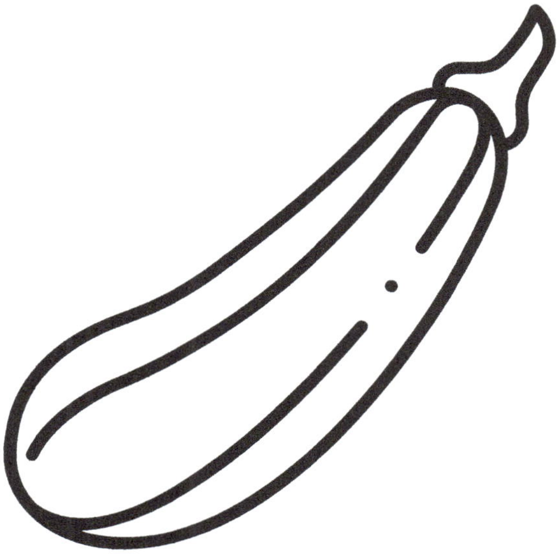

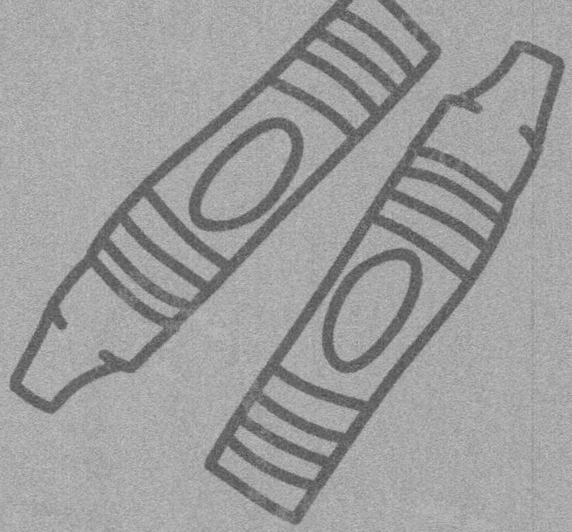

LEARNING ACTIVITIES

Fun and healthy learning activities!

COLOR THE ROOT VEGETABLES

These vegetables are grown underground because they are the root of the plant. For each of these vegetables, the plant stem and leaves are seen above ground!

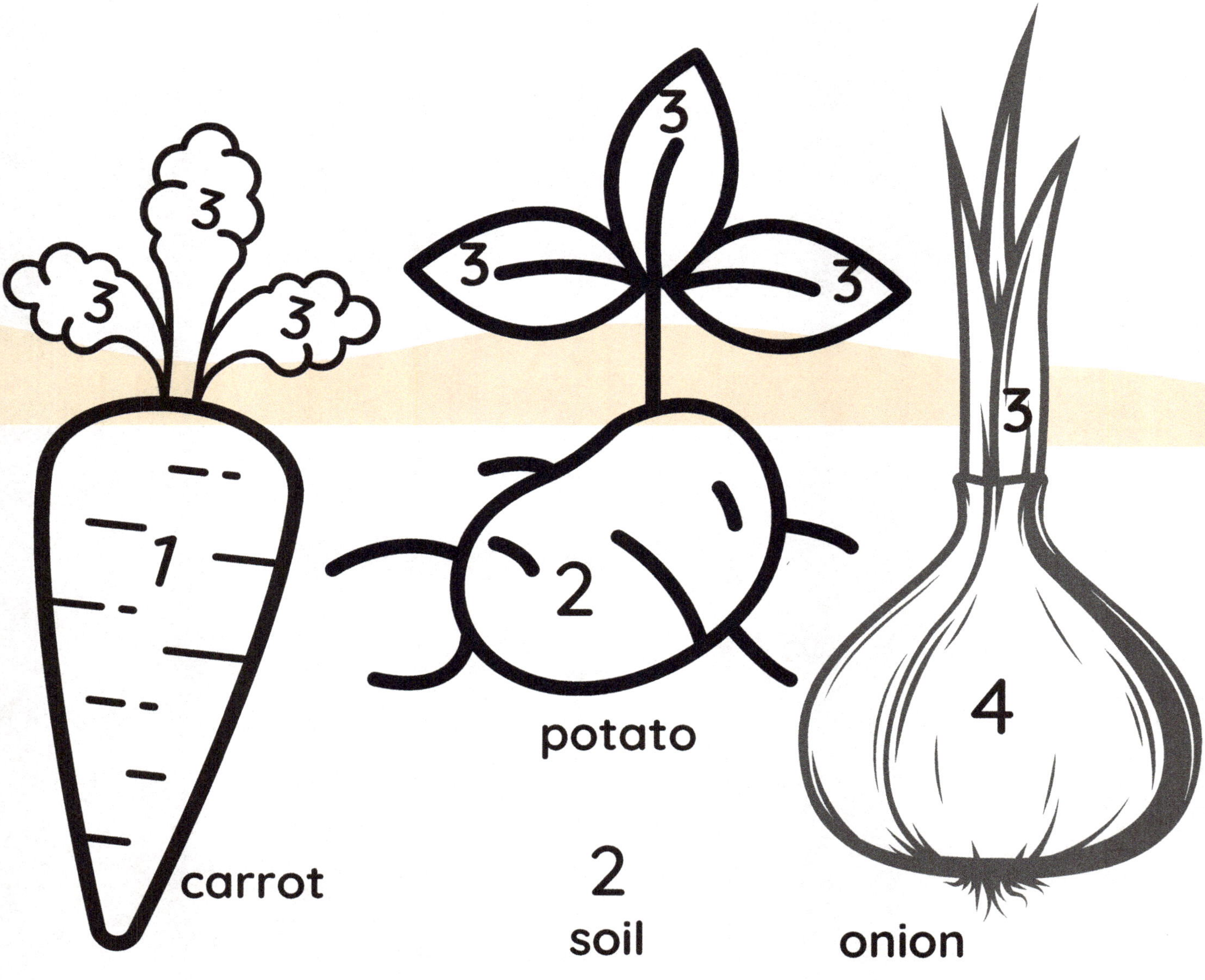

Color 1: orange
Color 2: brown
Color 3: green
Color 4: yellow

COLOR THE VINE PLANTS

These fruits & vegetables grow on vine plants! Examples of vine plants include melons, grapes, and squash!

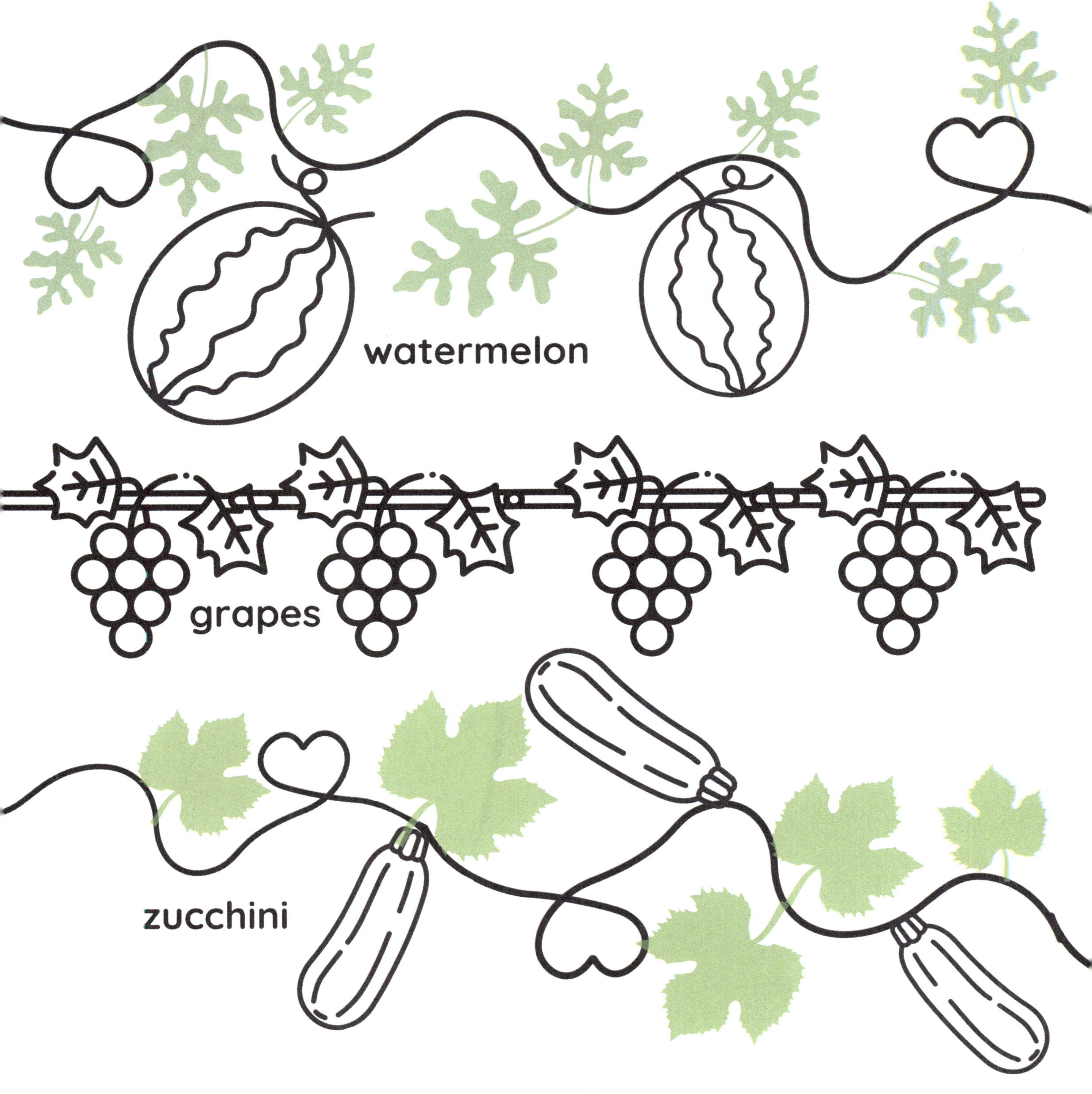

COLOR THE APPLE TREE

These fruits grow on trees. The apples grow out of flowers blossoms before turning into this delicious fruit.

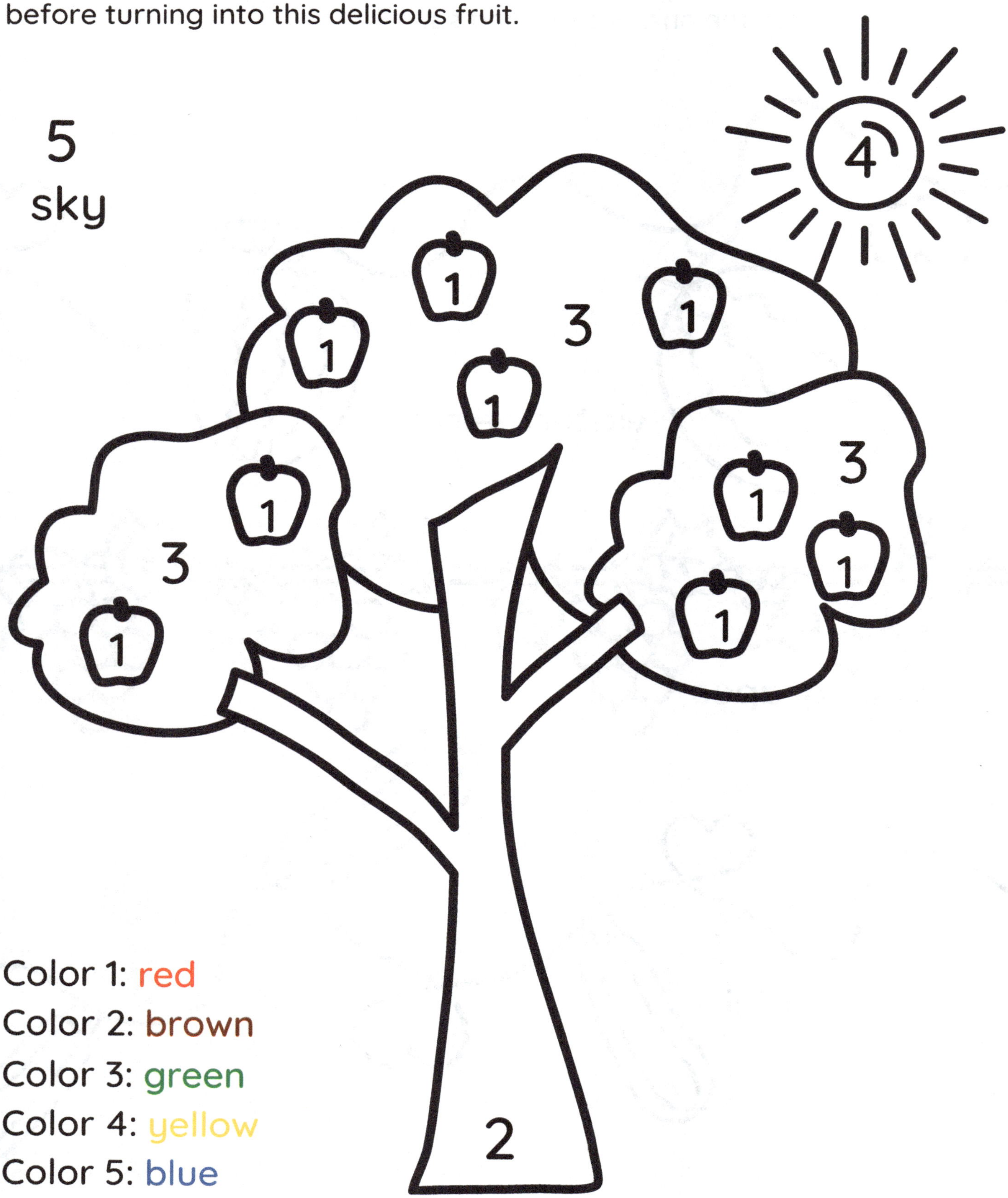

Color 1: red
Color 2: brown
Color 3: green
Color 4: yellow
Color 5: blue

COLOR YOUR PLATE!

Directions: Color the fruits and vegetables on the plate. For a healthy eating habit, eat fruits and vegetables from all different colors of the rainbow!

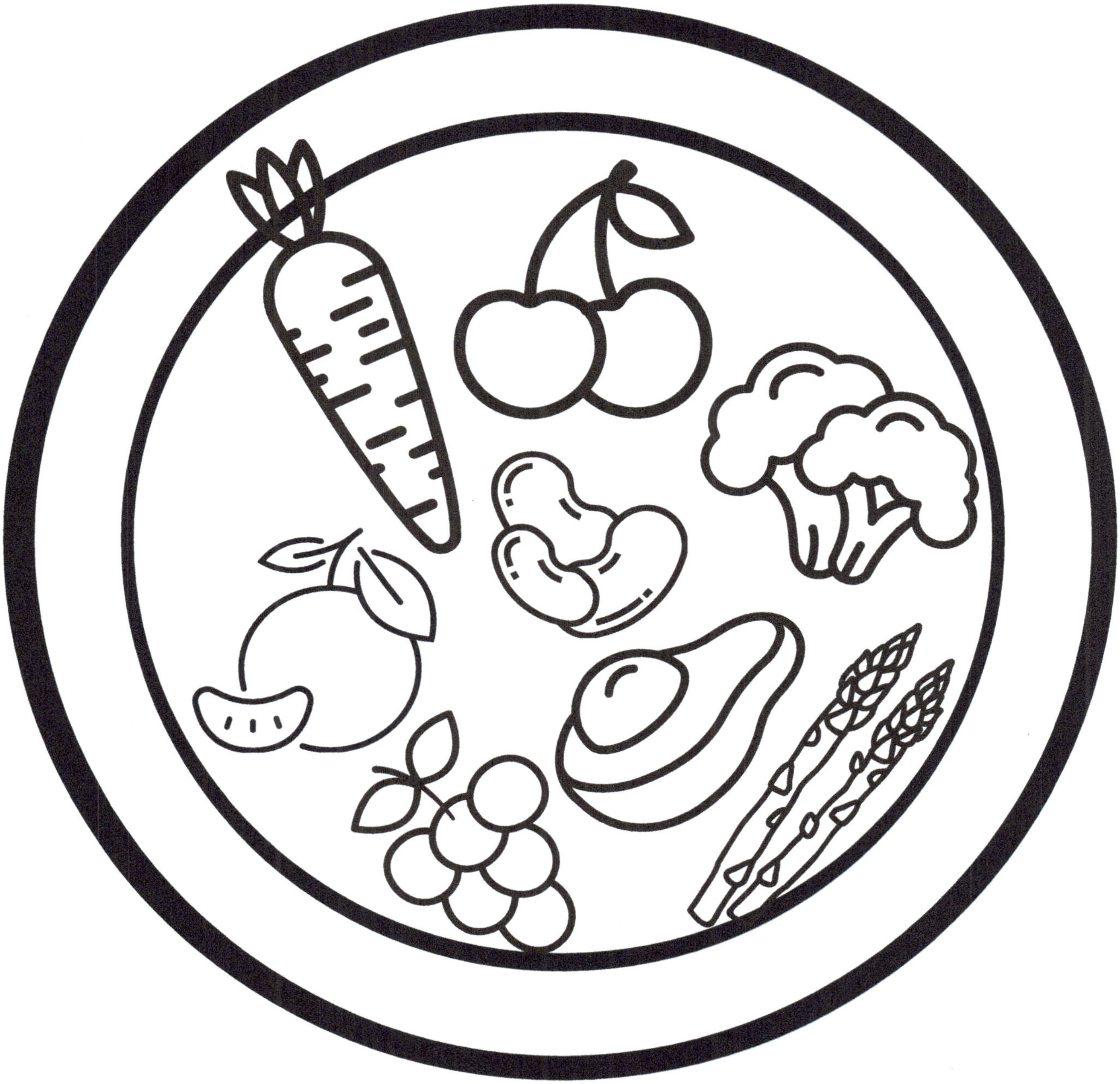

Bonus activity: Have your child find fruits and vegetables at home and place them all on a plate. Identify which ones are fruits vs. vegetables. Encourage them to hold each one and explore them using their five senses. Ask them about different ways they can eat this fruit or vegetable. Do they like it better raw, cooked, or in sauce form (like tomato sauce)? Which ones have they had before and which ones are new?

GUESS THE COLOR!

Directions: Identify the common color of all these fruits and vegetables. Once you've guessed it, color them that color!

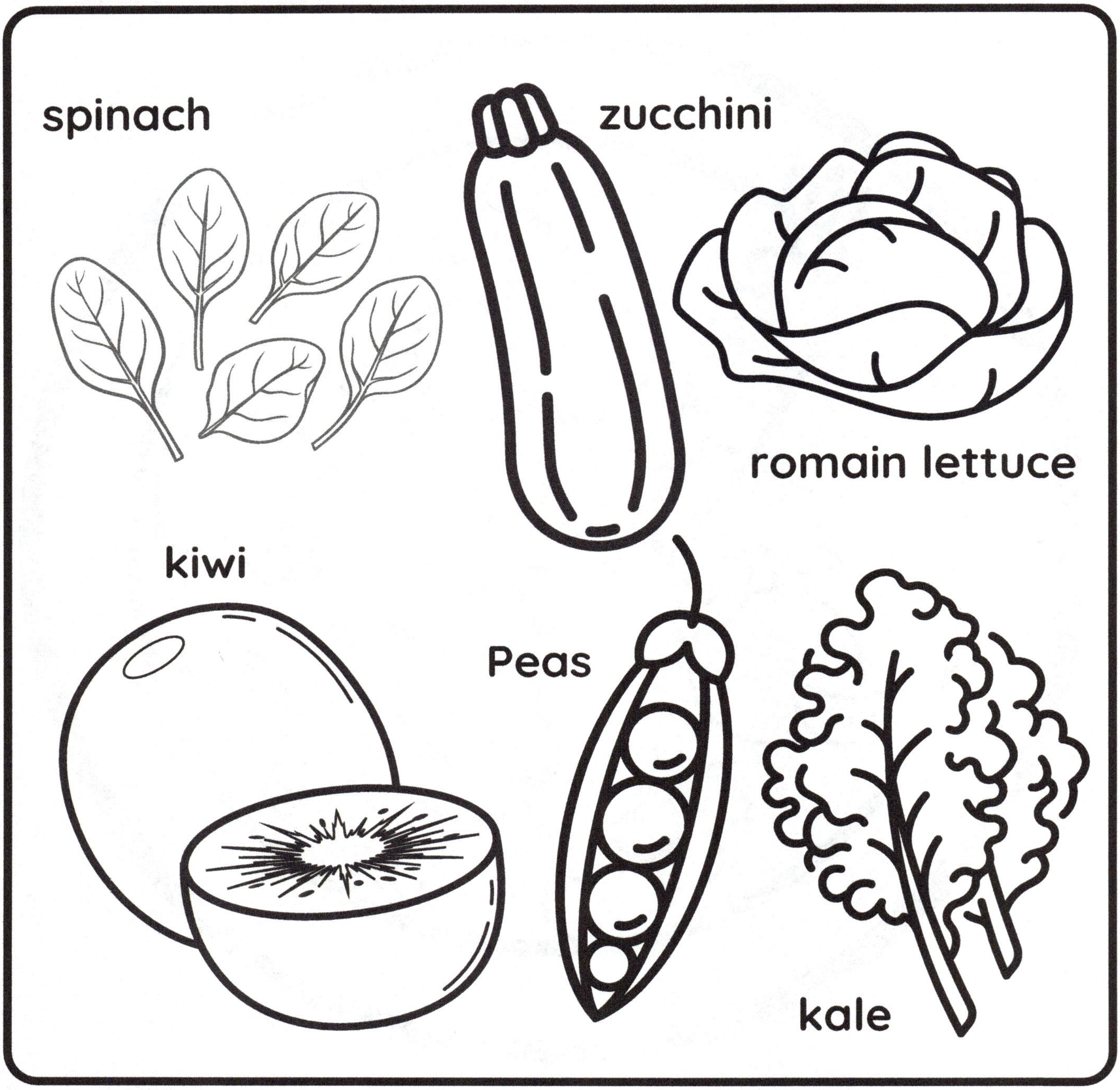

Bonus activity: A playful way to introduce new foods to your child is by serving them prepared foods in a muffin tin instead of a plate. Have your child explore the kitchen to find four different green foods including at least one new fruit or vegetable and one safe food. Examples include guacamole, celery with pesto dip, pea soup, etc. With each food placed in the muffin tin, encourage them to use their five senses with each one. Which one(s), if any, do they like today? Refer to "Introducing New Foods" in the Parent Guide for more tips!

GUESS THE COLOR!

Directions: Identify the common color of all these fruits and vegetables. Once you've guessed it, color them that color!

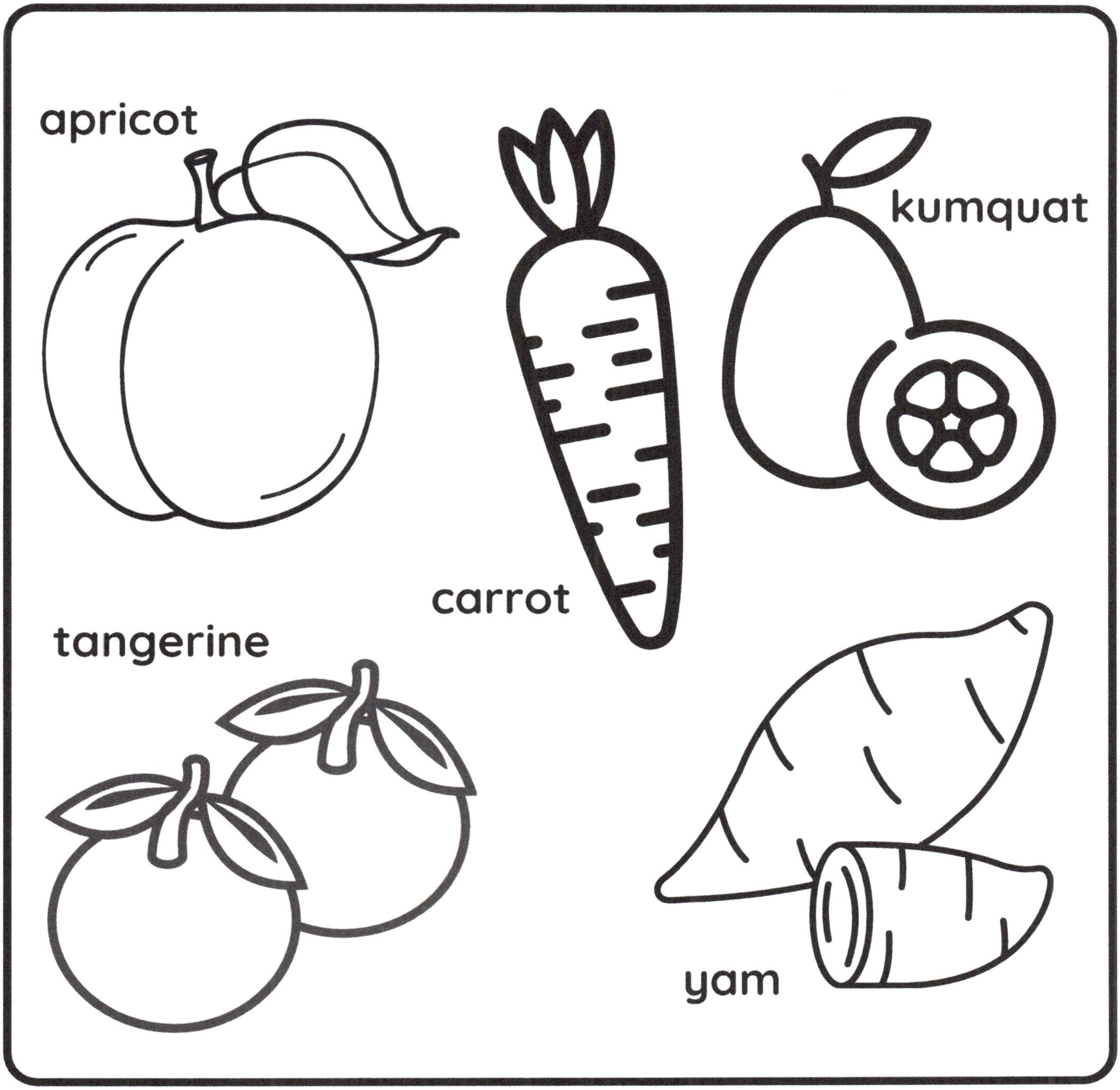

Bonus activity: Have your child explore the kitchen to find four different orange foods including at least one new fruit or vegetable and one safe food. Examples include orange slices, apricot jam, sweet potato fries, etc. With each food placed in the muffin tin, encourage them to use their five senses with each one. Which one(s), if any, do they like today? Refer to "Introducing New Foods" in the Parent Guide for more tips!

GUESS THE COLOR!

Directions: Identify the common color of all these fruits and vegetables. Once you've guessed it, color them that color!

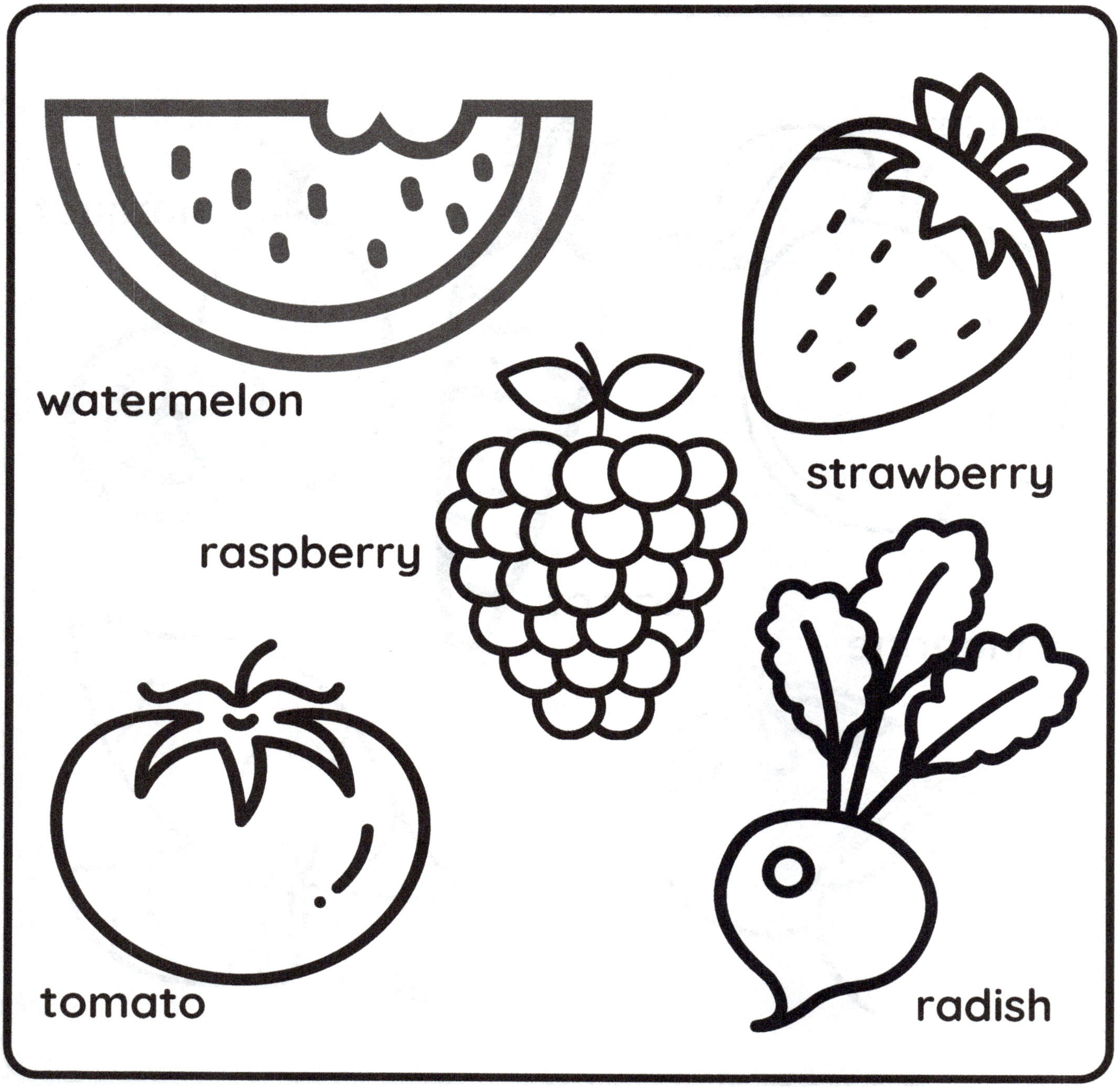

Bonus activity: Have your child explore the kitchen to find four different red foods including at least one new fruit or vegetable and one safe food. Examples include tomato soup, red fruit snacks, watermelon, etc. With each food placed in the muffin tin, encourage them to use their five senses with each one. Which one(s), if any, do they like today? Refer to "Introducing New Foods" in the Parent Guide for more tips!

GUESS THE COLOR!

Directions: Identify the common color of all these fruits and vegetables. Once you've guessed it, color them that color!

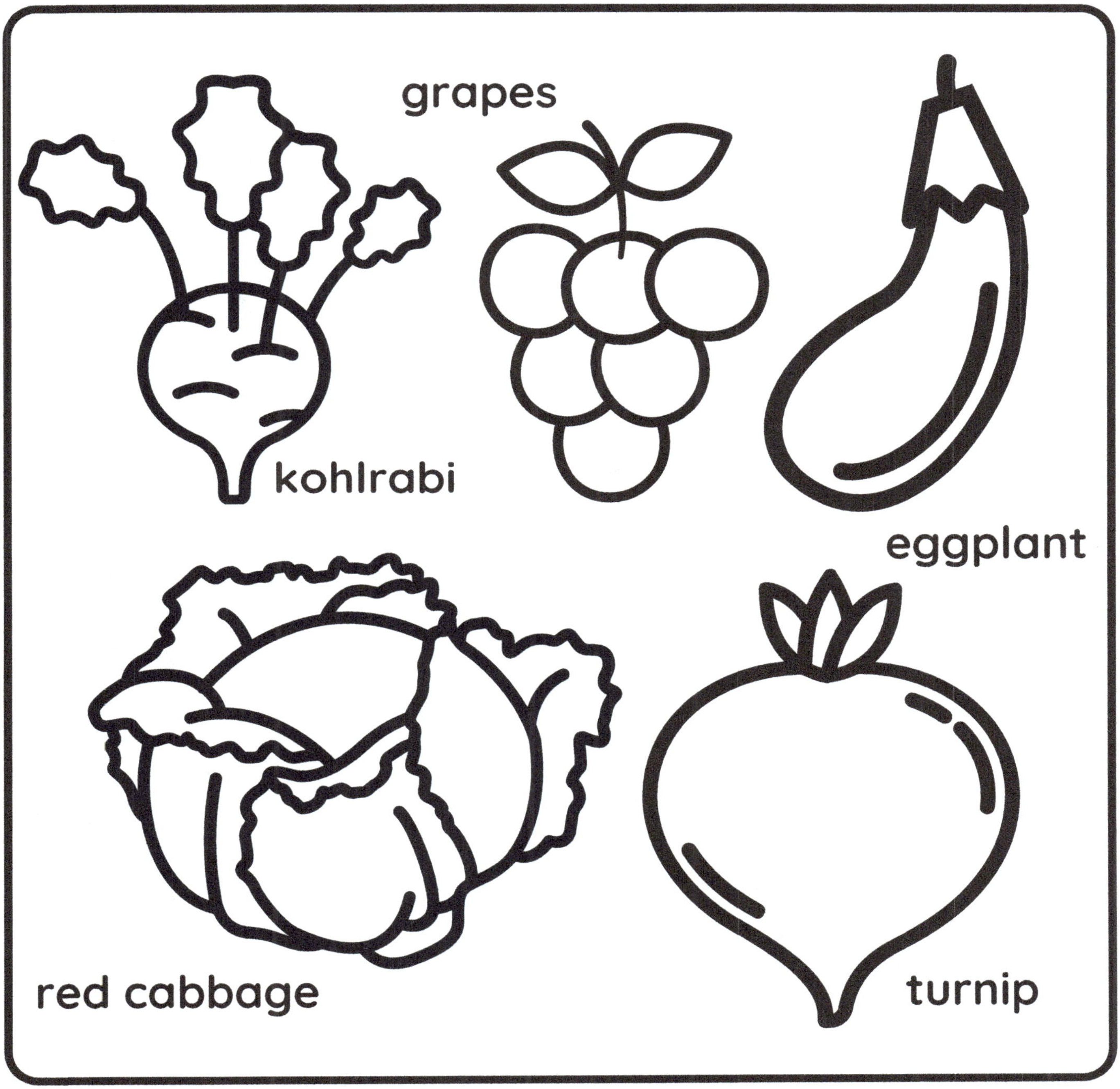

Bonus activity: Have your child explore the kitchen to find four different purple foods including at least one new fruit or vegetable and one safe food. Examples include red sauerkraut, grapes, purple carrot sticks, etc. With each food placed in the muffin tin, encourage them to use their five senses with each one. Which one(s), if any, do they like today? Refer to "Introducing New Foods" in the Parent Guide for more tips!

GUESS THE COLOR!

Directions: Identify the common color of all these fruits and vegetables. Once you've guessed it, color them that color!

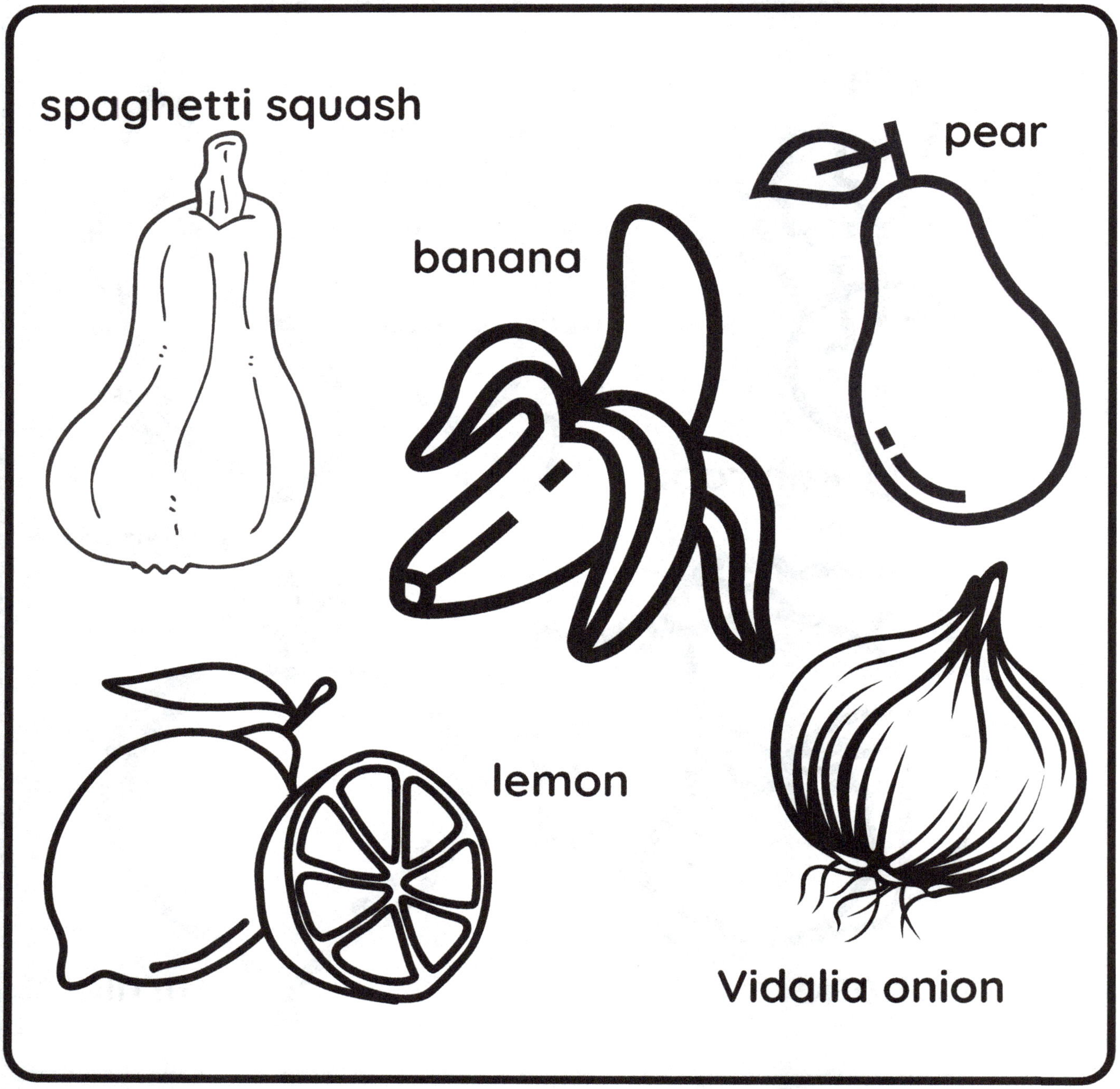

Bonus activity: Have your child explore the kitchen to find four different yellow foods including at least one new fruit or vegetable and one safe food. Examples include butternut squash soup, pear slices, lemon bar, etc. With each food placed in the muffin tin, encourage them to use their five senses with each one. Which one(s), if any, do they like today? Refer to "Introducing New Foods" in the Parent Guide for more tips!

TO-DO ACTIVITIES

Directions: Follow the dotted line to all these activities that are designed to get your child up and moving! Mark an 'X' next to the activities you complete. Have fun!

Take a walk around your neighborhood. Collect rocks, sticks, flowers and leaves. Use them to make words!

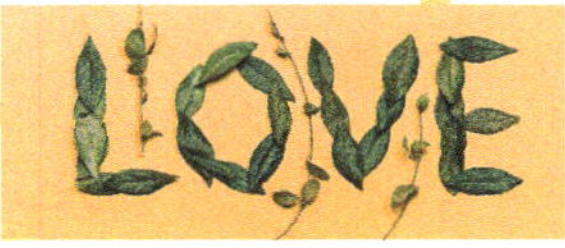

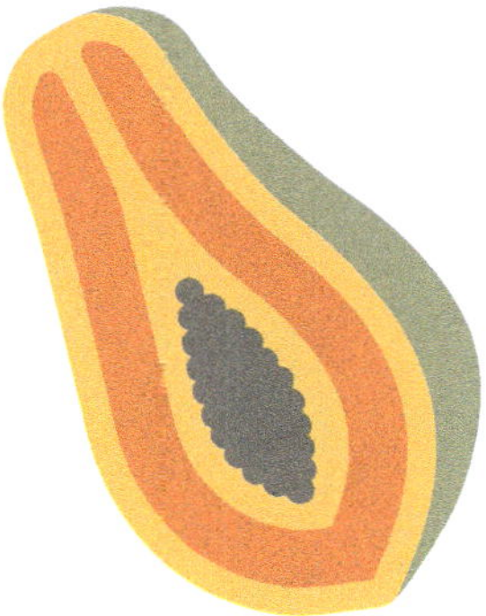

Take an alphabet walk. Pick any letter of the alphabet and find 10 things that start with that letter. Draw the things you found! Play again with a different letter.

Keep a journal with pictures or words of your favorite fruits and vegetables. Find more recipes to try and add them to the journal.

Pick a recipe with an adult and cook it together. Try out something new!

Adults: Great time to tie in measurement math lessons while cooking!

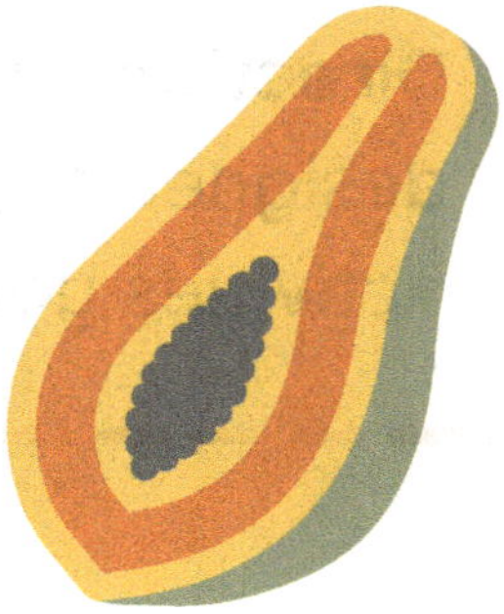

Go to the local farmer's market or grocery store with an adult and pick out a new fruit or vegetable that you have never tried.

Go outside and paint a picture of what nature you see!

When you're at the grocery store pick a color. Make a list of how many foods you can find in that color. Bonus point for every fruit and vegetable you find!

Shape Scavenger Hunt.
Pick a shape, and go on a walk. Find 5 things that have that shape. Draw what you find! Repeat with another shape.

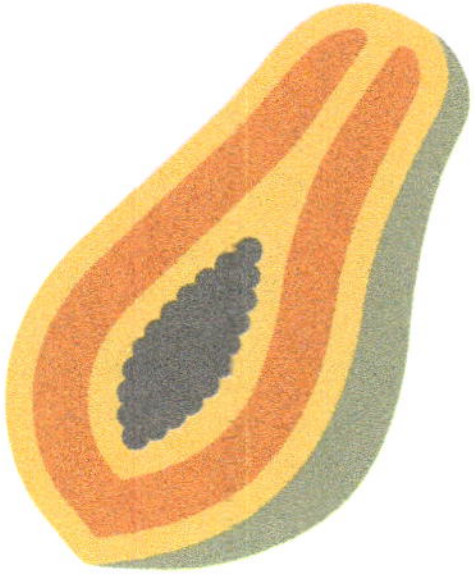

Color Scavenger Hunt.
Pick a color, and go on a walk. Find 5 things that have that color. Draw what you find! Repeat with another color.

Help plan dinners for the week with at least one new recipe that the family will like.

Leaf Prints.
Collect leaves outside. Lightly paint the leaf and stamp onto paper.

Plant a garden. Start with a list of tools and materials. Write out a schedule for watering and maintenance. Keep a journal with words and pictures to track progress.

Awesome job! You completed all the activities!

RECIPES

Healthy kid-friendly meal and snack ideas!

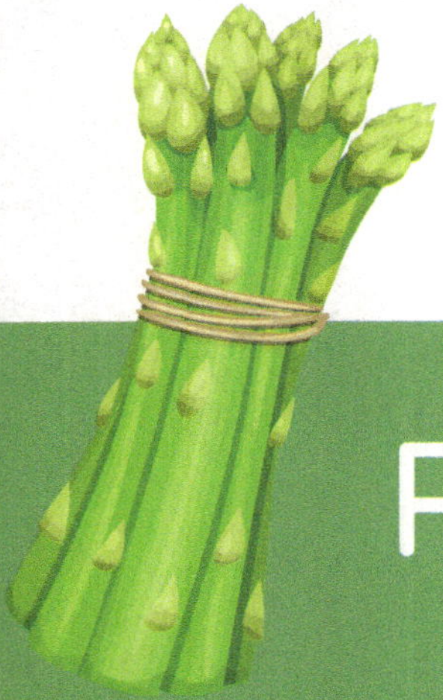

ASPARAGUS

Pasta Salad with Asparagus

Serves 6

INGREDIENTS

1 lb pasta (spiral or bowtie)

1 cup asparagus cut into 1 inch pieces

2 cups vegetables of choice (bell peppers, cherry tomatoes, cucumbers, celery, etc.)

1 can (2.25 oz) sliced black olives, drained

Italian dressing

1 Tbsp olive oil

INSTRUCTIONS

1. Cook pasta al dente. Rinse under cold water and drain.
2. Sauté asparagus with olive oil in frying pan for 10 mins or until tender to fork. Let cool.
3. Cut up vegetables of choice into bite-sized pieces.
4. In a salad bowl, combine the pasta, vegetables, asparagus, and olives. Pour dressing over salad. Toss and refrigerate overnight.

BLUEBERRY

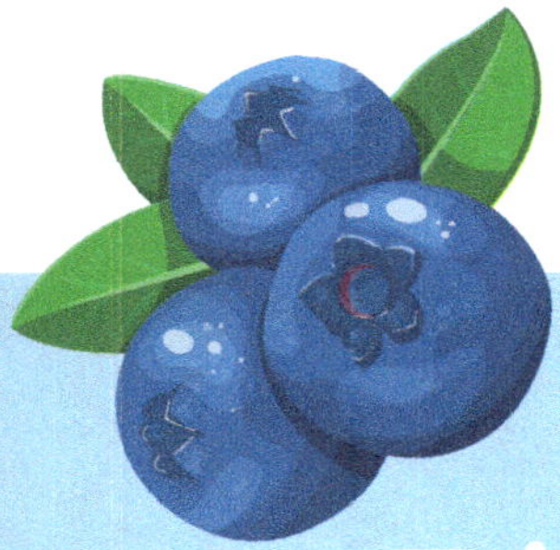

Blueberry Smoothie

Serves 1-2

INGREDIENTS

1 cup frozen blueberries

1 banana

1/2 cup Greek yogurt (flavor of choice)

1/4 cup almond milk (or milk of choice)

1/2 cup water

INSTRUCTIONS

1. Blend all ingredients together in a blender. Add ice or more frozen blueberries to thicken the smoothie; add more liquid to thin the smoothie.

CELERY

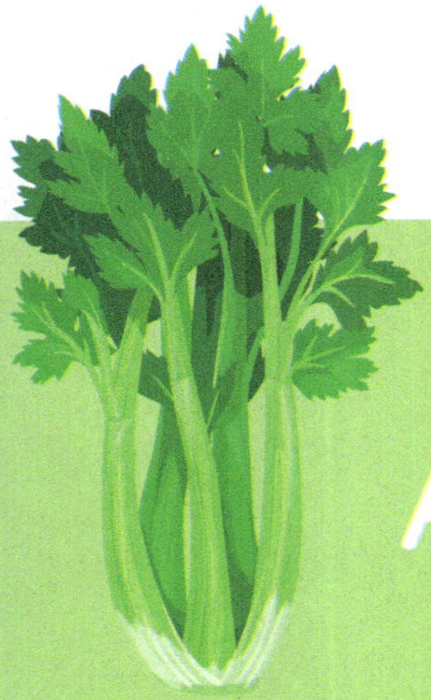

Ants on a Log

INGREDIENTS

Celery

Nut Butter
(peanut, almond,
sunflower, etc...)

Raisins

INSTRUCTIONS

1. Cut celery stocks into 3-4 inch sticks.
2. Fill celery with nut butter of choice.
3. Sprinkle raisins (the "ants") onto the celery "logs".

DATES

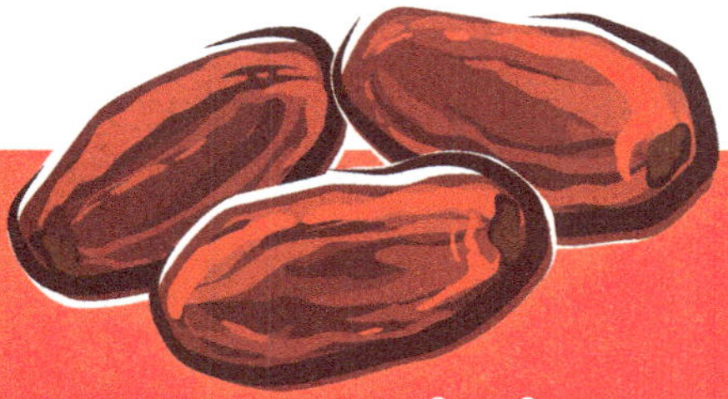

Nut Butter Dates

INGREDIENTS

Pitted dates

Favorite nut butter (peanut, almond, sunflower, etc...)

INSTRUCTIONS

1. Make a slit in the pitted date (be careful not to cut it in half).
2. Fill date with your favorite nut butter.
3. Optional: Add toppings of choice, such as cinnamon, crumbled nuts, coconut, sesame seeds...

JICAMA

Jicama Sticks & Dip

INGREDIENTS

Jicama

Favorite dip or guacamole

INSTRUCTIONS

1. If jicama is whole, peel then cut into strips (1/4 inch wide, 3 inches long. Or, you can purchase pre-cut jicama sticks.
2. Dip your crunchy jicama sticks into your favorite dip, like ranch dressing or guacamole!

KALE

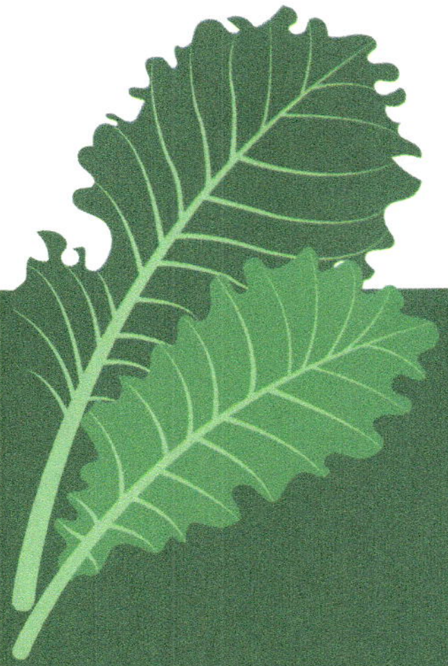

Kale Chips

Serves 2

INGREDIENTS

1 bunch of kale (about 4 cups)

2 tablespoon olive oil

1/4 teaspoon sea salt & spices of choice (such as pepper, chili powder, parmesan cheese)

INSTRUCTIONS

1. Preheat oven to 375°F.
2. Chop kale into bite-sized pieces then place them in a large bowl.
3. Drizzle olive oil over the kale leaves then mix with your hands until the kale is evenly coated in oil. Sprinkle with seasonings of choice.
4. Bake for 10 mins (or until crispy) on parchment-lined baking sheets. Serve immediately.

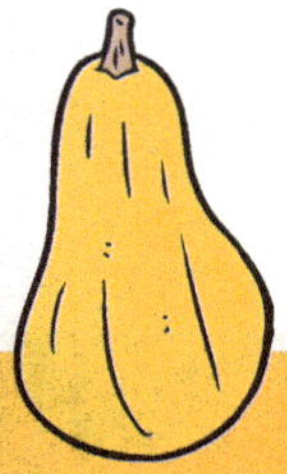

SPAGHETTI SQUASH

Cheesy Spaghetti Squash Casserole

Serves 4

INGREDIENTS

1 spaghetti squash, 3 lbs.

1/2 cup plain Greek yogurt

1/2 cup cheddar cheese

1/2 cup grated parmesan

1 egg

1 Tbsp minced garlic

1 tsp salt

1/2 tsp thyme

1/2 tsp black pepper

INSTRUCTIONS

1. Cut squash in half and scrape the seeds out.
2. Bake squash on a lightly greased baking pan for 45 mins at 400°F. When done, use a fork to scrape out the inside of the squash (it will look like noodles). Place these "noodles" into a lightly greased casserole pan.
3. In a mixing bowl, lightly whisk the egg. Mix in the yogurt, garlic, cheeses, and seasonings.
4. Pour mixture over "noodles" and stir until the squash is coated.
5. Bake for 40 mins.

VALENCIA ORANGE

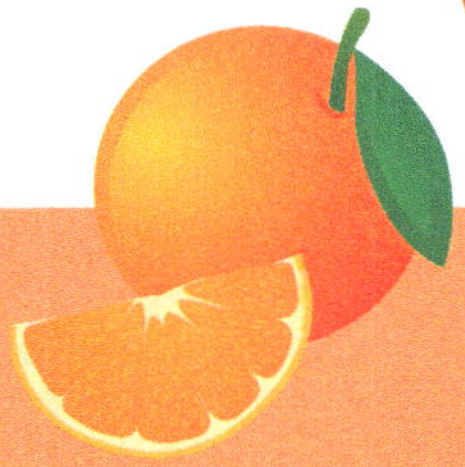

Orange Juice Popsicles

INGREDIENTS

6-7 Valencia oranges

10 wooden popsicle sticks

INSTRUCTIONS

1. Cut oranges in half.
2. Juice the oranges using a hand-held juicer.
3. Pour the juice in popsicle mold (should yield around ten 2.5 oz popsicles) and insert wooden sticks.
4. Freeze for 4-5 hours and enjoy!

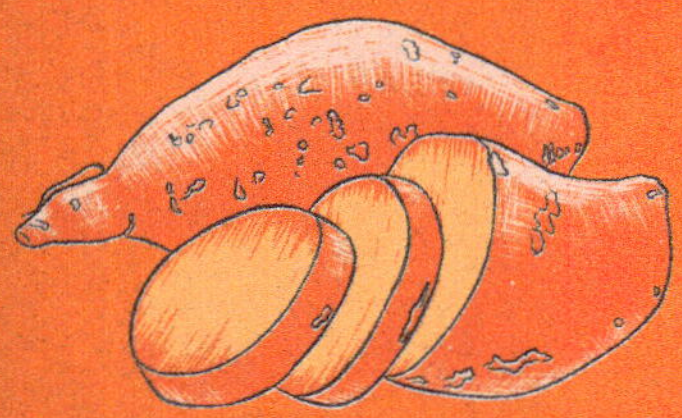

Sweet Potato (Yam) Fries

Serves 4

INGREDIENTS

2 lbs. yams or sweet potatoes

1/4 cup olive oil

2 Tbsp parsley

Spices of choice

INSTRUCTIONS

1. Preheat oven to 400°F.
2. Cut potatoes into strips (1/4 inch wide, 3 inches long).
3. Mix olive oil & spices into a bowl.
4. Place potato strips onto a baking sheet. Drizzle olive oil mixture over the potatoes and mix with hands until evenly coated.
5. Bake for 25-30 mins.
6. Top with finely chopped parsley and serve with your favorite dip.

ZUCCHINI

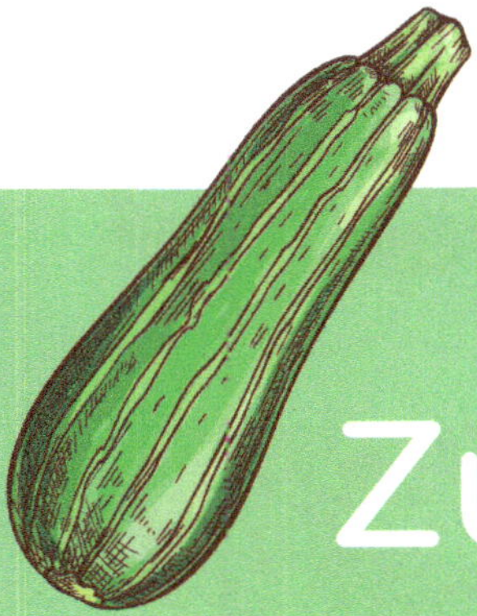

Zucchini Boat Pizza

Serves 4

INGREDIENTS

3 whole large zucchinis

1 lb ground turkey

Olive oil

Marinara sauce

Shredded mozzarella cheese

INSTRUCTIONS

1. Preheat oven to 375°F.
2. Cut zucchini in half (length-wise) & scrape the seeds out to make a "boat".
3. Cook ground turkey in a skillet.
4. Layout cut zucchini onto a lightly greased baking sheet.
5. Fill zucchini with layered marinara sauce and cooked turkey meat. Top with cheese.
6. Bake for 15-20 mins.

HAVE YOU TRIED IT?

- [ ] asparagus
- [ ] blueberries
- [ ] jicama
- [ ] avocado
- [ ] figs
- [ ] kohlrabi
- [ ] lemon
- [ ] watermelon
- [ ] mango
- [ ] kiwi
- [ ] spinach
- [ ] kale
- [ ] apricot
- [ ] green beans
- [ ] strawberry
- [ ] zucchini
- [ ] cherry
- [ ] lima beans

CHALLENGE: TRY SOMETHING NEW!

Made in the USA
Monee, IL
02 November 2026

67384187R00052